Since you communicated [...] which would not go away [...] completely cleared up and has never come back. I can't thank you enough for your assistance with Bella and for opening my mind to what is really possible.

Avril Norman, NSW, Australia

After a consultation with Trisha I started her technique of talking to Monty and using visualisation to send messages to him. Literally overnight he became much calmer and seemed happier. I now feel that he is closer than ever to me as we have connected on a different level.

Charmayne, NSW, Australia

Trisha chatted with Rafik, my Saluki dog, and shared with me what he was feeling and trying to tell me. Those wise words from my dog totally transformed the way I interact with him and all my animal companions.

Max Webb, dog groomer, WA, Australia

In desperation about the constant bloodied remains of some unidentifiable rodent all over my living room carpet, delivered by my cat Apollo, the Universe took pity on me in the form of Trisha McCagh. After her consultation the results were immediate. No more carcasses.

Barry Eaton, radio presenter, NSW, Australia

This has got to be one of the most incredible things that I have ever had the good fortune to experience. Everything that I had suspected about Bones my lion was actually put into words. Having an insight into how he is feeling has been tremendously helpful. You have no idea how grateful I am.

Roxy, Zimbabwe, Africa

The result from Trisha communicating with my cat Kenjiro was amazing. She was able to get all the information I had asked about, which gave me greater understanding of his needs and about his past. This created a closer bond in our relationship and so I am extremely grateful to Trisha for this.

Alice Wolf, Neu-Isenburg, Germany

After the sudden death of my husband, I was left with a traumatised cat that would not respond to love and had severe weight loss. After my consultation with Trisha, within 24 hours, in he came, tail up, hungry, chatting, and we have never looked back. I am eternally grateful as I could not bear to lose him as well.

Yvonne Ferrell, internationally renowned psychic,
West Sussex, England

STORIES FROM

The Animal
Whisperer

What your pet is thinking
and trying to tell you

TRISHA McCAGH

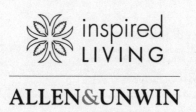

inspired
LIVING

ALLEN&UNWIN

Allen & Unwin
83 Alexander Street
Crows Nest NSW 2065
Australia
Phone: (61 2) 8425 0100
Fax: (61 2) 9906 2218
Email: info@allenandunwin.com
Web: www.allenandunwin.com

Cataloguing-in-Publication details are available from the National Library of Australia
www.librariesaustralia.nla.gov

ISBN: 978 1 74175 950 1 (pbk.)

Typeset in Australia by Bookhouse in 11.5/15 pt Bembo
Printed in Australia by McPherson's Printing Group

10 9 8 7 6 5 4 3 2

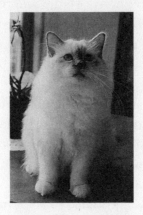

I dedicate this book in the memory of my beloved cat Beau, who without our magical meeting it would never have come into existence. He took me on a journey of self-discovery and expansive insights into the amazing world of animals. Beau showed me a depth of unconditional love I had never experienced before, and his divine guidance put me on the path that was to be my mission. He taught me to trust and believe in my dreams. His words, 'When everything is perfect nothing grows', continually shapes my outlook that life is a myriad of twists and turns in an on-going learning process.

Mattie, an exquisite and beautiful birman cat, became my supreme teacher and gave me the guidance, encouragement and the confidence I needed in my early days and beyond in my quest to be the voice of the animals. She is both my beloved best friend and mentor. Shea, an extremely handsome male birman cat with a lion's heart, has always been my pillar of support, providing me with the courage and strength to move continually forward on my life's journey. Shea's devotion and endless love has truly brought me to a special place in my heart. Mattie and Shea have together assisted me in holding animal communication in the highest esteem and the integrity it deserves. Being able to hear the words and wisdom of the animals is the ultimate in joy and enrichment of the heart.

Akeira and Savannah, my beloved Japanese Spitz dogs, put the word 'fun' into my world. They make me feel childlike again and I experience pure joy in my heart when I need it most. Life is always filled with extreme excitement and optimism when we are together.

This book is also dedicated to all of my beloved animals who have shared and given me so many life-changing experiences. Their amazing understanding along with unconditional love and support has helped to shape me into the person I am today. Special thanks to Slasher, Cimmeron, Winston and Misty.

A special thanks also to all the animals on the planet. They have enriched so many lives and taught us to live harmoniously and to love unconditionally to create a perfect world. Dreams really do come true.

Contents

Part IV: Animals Are Not Human

Part V: Breeders and Pet Shops

Part VI: Competitive Arenas

Part VII: Respecting the Natural World

Prologue

BELIEVE IT OR NOT, ANIMALS ARE JUST LIKE US IN SO MANY WAYS. They have a sense of humour. They hurt. They get confused, unhappy, depressed. They need love and attention, to feel part of their human family, to be included and respected. Once you start to understand the intricacies of the animal world, your life and theirs will never be the same. I know, because that is what happened to me.

You picked up this book because you care about animals. You have a hunch that they can communicate, but don't understand how. You are right, they can communicate. The more you 'get' them, the more you will be able to pick up on what they are trying to say to you.

My love affair with animals started when I was growing up. I lived with my parents and two sisters. My father was involved in livestock, travelling long distances to rural areas. During school holidays and weekends I'd go with him. If I wasn't doing that, I'd be spending the day with our animals. There were always dogs, cats and birds in abundance at home. I'm from a long line of animal lovers, from my great-grandparents to my present clan. I honestly can't remember a time without at least one animal around.

Above all else, I had an absolute affinity to horses. They reminded me of the strength and freedom in us all that are waiting to be unleashed. When other kids were watching television or playing with their friends, I was usually in the backyard, neighing and galloping around like a horse. And I wasn't content just to be able to ride them; I wanted to experience the entire essence of what it was like to be a horse. In my mind, *I* was a horse, and mesmerised by anything that resembled one.

I had what I discovered was an amazing gift. I could 'see' through the eyes of animals and communicate with them as if I was one. Luckily for me I wasn't institutionalised, just a bit misunderstood!

Just to explain: I get this communication from animals in many ways. I *hear* the words, animal speak, in my mind, and I also get a lot of visuals, either in single pictures or like a 'video'. The message they're trying to get across comes to me telepathically. I can also feel their emotions in my body. Plus I have the added power of being intuitive, and this kicks in as well. I call this skill 'pure knowing'. With all these images and impressions I can build up an accurate picture of what is going on with the animal.

Hey, I know this sounds crazy, but it's real. And what makes it even more amazing is that I'm just a girl from the suburbs, and not the only one out there with such a great love of animals. But I am someone who felt so compelled by my feelings that I decided to do something about it. I learnt to listen to animals deeply and carefully with my heart, and what I've discovered has taken me on this amazing journey.

In a lifetime of loving animals, and through my many years working as an animal whisperer, I've learnt that there is nothing more wonderful than sharing your life with animals. But this only works when they are happy. Sometimes we have to make the effort to find out what they want, and what they need, in order for them to be contented. That's where I come in, and *you* can learn the secret too.

There were many animals who were very special to me when I was growing up, including a thoroughbred called Ali Baba. He lived with an old friend of my father's, who ran a riding school. This friend agreed to let me ride Ali Baba some weekends. Ali, as I called him, was an extremely regal horse, tall in stature, a rich brown colour, and very handsome. He was an ex-trotter, so trotting was the style he felt most comfortable doing with me on board. He was very confident and determined in his approach, always felt in complete control on our rides and was ever protective of those in his care.

I was ten at the time and while I rode him I'd tell him about my problems, day-to-day activities, and about what I wanted to do when I grew up. After speaking with him I'd feel relieved, as I knew he understood. He always made me feel important. He was so patient and such an intent listener. I'd watch his ears turn back toward me as I spoke, and his trotting would change rhythm, depending on the tone of my voice. In fact, I knew Ali understood me far better than anyone else. It was very consoling to me as a young girl.

In many instances my animal family became my best friends. During times of hardship in my human family, I'd turn to my animal friends for comfort and support. Many of you will know exactly what I'm talking about when I refer to being a small child in a household where bad things are going on between the adults in the home. I've never really talked about this until now, but somehow it finally feels okay to open up on such a dark topic in order to describe how animals were my salvation. You're powerless and you're scared, and you look for ways to find reassurance. For me it was my darling animals who loved me unconditionally and wouldn't have known how to be cruel. It was something I could rely on, and this certainty continued into my adult years.

I guess what I'm saying is: never underestimate the healing power of snuggling up to a much-loved pet.

When I finished high school I went to university, graduating as a dental hygienist and working at that career for many years. Although I enjoyed the challenge, I always felt deep down that something was missing.

People often commented on how intuitive I was, but at that stage I wasn't taking it too seriously. That was until the day when I had this deep knowing that I was to leave my place of birth and travel to the other side of the country. It's hard to explain, but there was a strong sensation in my gut that there'd be change; a feeling that couldn't be ignored, because it wouldn't go away.

I knew the move was part of the bigger picture of my life, and that this shift in location was a necessity. I'm sure we all get these intuitive signs from time to time, but acting on them is the crucial difference. It definitely raised a few eyebrows when I told my family I was about to leave not only them, but also my highly paid, successful position in dentistry, as well as rent out my house and place all my belongings in storage to relocate to a city a thousand kilometres away.

As the day to leave neared, my family and friends grew to accept the idea and became excited for me. So I boarded the flight with two bags of clothes and was off to the unknown.

Within two weeks of arriving in the Big Smoke, I was sharing an apartment, had secured a job and made a couple of new friends. Everything seemed to be going according to a plan—although it wasn't a conscious plan, if you know what I mean.

After a few months, I was settled in and enjoying my new life. I felt I had taken on a new identity and was free to choose any path I wanted. One night I was invited to a party by some friends and it was there I met the man of my dreams, Peter.

After a relatively short courtship, he and I married, and we settled down happily together. However, content as I was with Peter, it wasn't long before I craved animal companions once more in my life. But, when I broached the subject of getting a kitten, Peter wasn't overly enthusiastic, although he certainly did not oppose the idea.

My husband is a kind, very social and laid-back person who somehow manages to create harmony wherever he goes. You can talk to him about anything, and he's open to new things. This meant he agreed we could go and look at kittens. I loved him for that. So we went off kitten hunting, and one of the first places we visited was the home of a lady named Deb, who had a litter of Birman kittens: three girls and two boys.

Straight away I noticed this tiny, angelic individual. Deb actually asked us to consider a boy kitten called Psycho Boy, who was full of life and very exciting, but I just couldn't take my eyes of this other little boy. I picked him up—and as our eyes met, my heart melted. He cuddled up into my neck and went to sleep.

We had other kittens to see that day so we told Deb we'd let her know. Even though we saw dozens of other gorgeous kittens, I just couldn't get my mind off that first little boy . . . so back we went and bought him, instantly naming him Beau. And Beau changed my life.

PART I

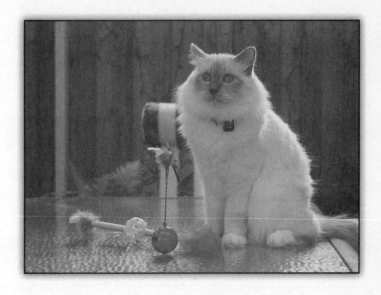

Listen and Learn

1

Beau: The Kitten that Changed My Life

BEAU WAS ONE OF THE SMALLEST IN THE LITTER AND, AFTER A week of leaving him on his own during the day while we worked, I decided he needed company. Peter and I again went to Deb to see if one of Beau's sisters was available, only to find they were all spoken for. While she made us a coffee, I couldn't resist getting down on the floor with the kittens and having fun. After a few minutes one little girl was desperately trying to get my attention, so I picked her up and she immediately fell asleep in my arms.

I asked if there was any chance the person due to take this cutie might change her mind. Deb said, 'No,' as the little kitten was being flown to Holland. So that looked like the end of it. I asked Deb to let us know if the situation changed. She said she would, but that it was unlikely. The strange thing, though, was that I still felt the female kitten was somehow going to be part of our family, and I had grown to trust my strong intuitive feelings.

Two days later Deb phoned and guess what? Her friend in Holland had just found out she was pregnant and therefore didn't wish to take on a kitten. If we still wanted her, she was ours! I was over there the next day to pick her up, quite delirious with happiness. I named her Mattie, and within a few days Mattie and Beau were inseparable.

Peter had never had cats before so this was a new experience for him, and he was so cute with the attention he gave them. For the first few weeks when I'd pick them up, I'd find they had wet paws. What was going on? I finally found out that Peter had been washing their paws every time they had gone to the kitty litter! And when we discovered Beau had had a back problem from birth, gorgeous Peter began building him a disabled ramp so he could climb up it to look out the window. I'll never forget Peter's sweetness and the way he embraced cats as part of our little family.

Tiny Beau grew into an absolute vision. He was gorgeous, as was Mattie, but Beau was unique. Every time he had a fur ball, or his food didn't agree with him, no matter where he was in the house, he'd run to the bathroom to be sick. Can you believe it?

Beau slept in the bed with us, but in the middle of the night he'd go over to the window and howl at the moon. I'm not kidding you. After a while it was such a usual occurrence, we hardly noticed it happening.

These two felines soon became a very big part of our lives, especially Beau, as he and I developed a special bond. Acquaintances and friends who saw us together invariably remarked that there was something different about our connection that they just couldn't put their finger on. I had a link with him that I hadn't experienced with any other animal. Actually, I felt like I'd known Beau before. We shared a bond I couldn't explain.

Beau was a very gentle and loving soul. He had a quiet demeanour and was never obtrusive. He was content to be close to me whenever I was at home and he'd groom me as if I was one of his offspring. He spent half an hour one day grooming my arm. Although slightly uncomfortable for me with his raspy tongue, it was such a beautiful gesture that I lay there and enjoyed his attention.

This little cat was so patient with every situation and created a remarkable calmness around me. He was very much an old soul, mature far beyond his months of life, who breathed a ray of sunshine into each and every day. Best of all, he brought out an inner beauty in me I'd never been aware of before.

We all have positives and negatives, but with Beau I only ever experienced positives. As unrealistic as it sounds, it was true. He showed me how to simply *be*, which is perhaps the greatest gift of all.

When Beau was thirteen months old, my whole world was rocked apart. One night we came home and, for once, he wasn't at the door to greet us. I immediately felt panic as I just knew something bad had happened.

I ran frantically around the apartment looking for him, and I finally saw him lying on the floor. He'd collapsed, his legs were rigid and he was dribbling from his mouth. My legs went weak and my heart was all-but beating out of my chest. I picked him up, placed him in his bed and raced off to the veterinary hospital in the car with Peter driving and me with Beau on my lap.

On the way I started to stroke his head, telling him not to worry, and that I'd look after him. All of a sudden he was calm and relaxed and just looking up at me, like he had everything under control. Then as we arrived at the vet he relapsed, and I was distraught.

The vet rushed Beau in and put him on life support. They carried out some tests and found he had a genetic disorder. He was having a metabolic shutdown. This couldn't be happening! The mere thought of anything more than the tiny back problem afflicting Beau was too painful for me to even imagine. Finally the vet said there was little hope.

For two days I didn't sleep or eat while his life hung in the balance. I refused to accept that he might die and at the vet's just sat for hours holding Beau's little paw in my hand. I told him to hang on and not to give up. Then, as I leant down and kissed the side of his face, I heard him say to me, *I have to go, you have to set me free.* Beau's words seemed to come out of thin air, but they were as clear as the light of day. My initial thought was, how could he be saying this. But I knew deep down that he was talking to me. Even though I so wanted Beau to make it, I couldn't ignore his last wish.

I felt my heart breaking as I gave the instruction to have him put down. As his body went limp, I continued holding him in my arms for an hour—or was it two? Time seemed to stand still. Somehow I knew and could feel that he was still around me.

I understood I couldn't stay with his body forever, so I finally let go and handed him to the vet for cremation. Then, as I was about to leave, I just sensed I had to go to Deb's house. It was one of those pure knowings again. Peter, who was with me at the time, said that he was too upset, and asked if we could go tomorrow. But I knew it had to be today, and that Mattie had to come with us.

When I told Deb what had happened to Beau, we cried together. Then all of a sudden a kitten, the image of Beau, appeared. He crawled up my leg and meowed as if to make sure he had my attention. Deb said, 'This is Beau's half-brother.' He had nearly been sold that day, but for some reason she refused to let him go. I couldn't believe my eyes, because he was so like Beau. Deb said she wanted us to have this kitten to help take away the shadows of grief. He just happened to be nine weeks old and ready for a new home. Another so-called coincidence.

Normally I wouldn't think of such a thing, as I hadn't had time to grieve. From previous experience this could take several years. But I knew from my inner intuition we had to take this kitten home that night, so we did, naming him Shea. I felt a certain amount of guilt getting this tiny, innocent kitten, as I was still grief-stricken for Beau, who of course could never be replaced. How could I give this kitten the love and attention he needed when I felt so shattered? But Shea was such a strong character and an absolute charmer, that in no time he had worked his way into my heart.

Then one night after only a couple of days with us, the most amazing thing happened: Shea acted out Beau's behaviour down to the last detail. This nine-week-old kitten went to the two front windows and, yes, you guessed it, he howled at the moon. Peter and I were speechless. It was surely Beau's way of letting us know he was around and okay, and that there shouldn't be any mistaking it was him sending the message.

Being left with so many unanswered questions, I immediately went to the internet to see if I could find out where animal spirits go, and soon discovered that we can indeed communicate with animals, alive or passed over. These websites described exactly what I had experienced that day at the vet's with Beau, when he explained he needed to go. It was incredible to discover we can have this level of communication with animals—and that there were other people already doing this. I wanted to know more. I just *had* to know more.

As I continued my research, I found that most of the animal communicators were in the United States. Perhaps they could tell me more about Beau? I decided to arrange a consultation. The communicator validated my belief that Beau, Mattie and Shea had drawn me to Deb's house, that Shea was a gift of love, and that Beau did in fact communicate with me that sad day while he was on life support. She repeated his exact words. I was in shock.

So I *could* hear animals 'talking'! It was unbelievably wonderful—yet surreal at the same time. I knew then and there my life was about to change forever.

Homelife went on, however, as it does. Then one night Beau came to me just as I was about to fall asleep. He told me it was time to walk away from dentistry and follow my chosen path, and he assured me he'd be there to guide me. Furthermore, he let me know he understood that my love for him was as strong as ever.

Was this magical or what? I was so very grateful to Beau, as I felt for the first time in my life I'd found some of the missing pieces. I knew that with this guidance I'd finally feel complete. As I was about to learn, more help would come to me through my animal spirit guides.

This is something we don't know much about in the West, but just as we have angels or other guides, there are animal spirit guides. They have an unbelievable amount of wisdom to share, and they help us connect with the animal kingdom, and guide us along our life's journey.

Lifelong animal spirit guides are usually wild animals, not domesticated. If they're domesticated, then they usually have a link to a wild counterpart. In my case, Beau was my link to wolf wisdom or wolf medicine as it's often called by American Indians and shamens of many countries.

Mind you, not all animal spirits are lifelong. Some stay with you through a period of several years and some no more than a day. They may be there to assist you through a particularly tough time in your life, or to be your teacher throughout your entire spiritual development.

The wolf is known to spiritualists as a teacher of ancient wisdom, which gave me much insight into my future work. The symbol of the wolf became a very important part of everything I've learnt since then.

After this incredible dream, I began to hear Mattie and Shea communicating with me, as if they'd always spoken to me. I started to realise that if I could hear Beau, Mattie and Shea, I must be able to hear other animals speak too.

What exactly was this type of communication and how did it work, I wondered. I wasn't sure. So, I began talking to every animal I came into contact with, to test my newfound ability. If I could hear animals, then I had to find out if they could hear me.

It was then I discovered that animal communication happens all the time. Unlike us, they communicate silently from one mind to another without the use of speech or gestures. Part of this incredible gift is the ability to hear, feel or see near and far.

Remarkably, I learnt to hear and talk to all species of animals. It was just a case of sending and receiving messages with my mind, and using my intuitive sensing. The thought transmissions I receive can come in the form of feelings, emotions, mental images, impressions, sensations or pure knowing. They're received directly from an animal. And as I began to talk to animals in this silent language, I discovered that they express the same feelings and emotions, and have individual personalities, just like we do. They are pure of thought and their love is unconditional.

I assure you, we're all born with this ability, but sadly we lose it along the way, sidetracked by other parts of life. But the lovely thing is that it's just a matter of putting in the time to relearn this beautiful skill. When we begin to verbalise in human language as young children, we forget the silent language we once had. Just like muscles waste away when we no longer use them, we lose this skill—but it can be revived.

Now I'm blessed to live between worlds, reconnecting humans with the natural world. So one part of me lives in the human realm and the other in the animal realm. Not bad for a girl from the suburbs.

2

In Tune with Animals

I'D LIKE TO EXPLAIN WHY I BELIEVE IT'S POSSIBLE FOR EVERY
ONE of us to reconnect to the natural world and why it's
important that we do. Although animals have always been a
part of human families, the number of animals has been very
much on the increase over recent years. Animal companions
have become, for many people, a necessary addition to the
human existence. Why?

Well, in a strange kind of way, it's not all that complicated
and it's something I've always felt and understood. More
people are choosing to live in domesticity with animals as
they find unconditional love, loyalty and stability in these
relationships. In our ever-changing world of uncertainty, it
is like a breath of fresh air. These are buddies we can rely
on and express our love for, and they never reject us or let
us down in any shape or form.

Animals are the bridge between us and the beauty of all
that is natural. They show us what's missing in our lives, and
how to love ourselves more completely and unconditionally.

They connect us back to who we are, and to the purpose of why we're here. The more you respect an animal's intelligence, engage in a conversation with them, and treat them as close friends, the more amazing their responses are. They have opinions and desires, just as we do, but this doesn't mean there are to be no boundaries. Instead, it throws up the concept that there are perhaps new alternatives to be considered. This is true of human relationships too.

If someone treats you as inferior or with a lack of respect, it's unlikely you'd want to form a relationship with him or her. However when you're valued for who you are, it's uplifting. It encourages you to spend as much time as possible in this supportive atmosphere. It makes sense!

You'll find that most animals will wish to develop closer relationships with you when they're approached from *their* level of awareness. This gives a whole new perspective of awareness of ourselves that we probably haven't experienced for a long time. When communicating with animals in this intuitive way, it tends to clear many of the blockages that may arise in human perceptions, such as our filters or agendas regarding not only animals, but the entire world.

This natural form of communication puts you back in connection with your inner self. It realigns you to who you are and what your purpose is, simply by removing the judgemental attitudes you may have acquired in the modern world. When you're able to get all the information by a two-way conversation, instead of a one-sided persepctive, it's amazing how perceptions are changed and solutions present themselves far more effectively. That is why in our human world so much emphasis is placed on communication. So why not with other species?

It's important to see that merely *observing* behaviour (whether with animals or humans) is greatly limiting, and can be misleading. Without finding underlying causes to an issue, you are only relating to a portion of the problem, and assuming the rest. We have learnt through the cultural differences between people, how important communication is in our development and evolution as a species. But the same progress can be made when addressing other species, especially those we closely interact with.

As this intuitive or telepathic language is universal, having been practiced between humans and animals for centuries, it does make sense that all beings are born to communicate and understand each other. Think about it: most young children experience telepathic communication with others of any species even before they learn a formal language. Once verbal communication is encouraged by adults, communication by direct thought is inhibited, and eventually forgotten. This is true in other societies too. For example, if a Spanish couple with young children migrate to an English-speaking country and don't continue speaking in their native tongue, then the youngsters won't be able to speak fluent Spanish in their teenage years.

There are many ways to relearn this intuitive ability. Being in a place of nature regularly, sharing your life with animals, and attending animal-communicating workshops are examples. These will all help to reconnect you with the natural world.

Animals are very willing to communicate with you telepathically. All that's needed is your intention to do so. By this I mean you're cultivating a quiet mind so they can reach you without the usual incessant chatter going on in your brain. When your mind is constantly occupied by mindless noise, an animal's message just can't get through.

Also, you must have an earnest desire to listen to what they want to say to you, and, believe me, it will come if you create the right environment. When they communicate their thoughts, your brain can instantly translate them into words. If the animals are sending a visual scene to your mind, then you can perceive and sense the sights, sounds, emotions and feelings in this scene, just as the animals are experiencing them. At other times they're giving you the sensations of emotion and feelings from *their* body to *your* awareness.

Looking beyond an animal's physical body and sensing their awareness, you will soon see their level of intelligence and depth of emotion. Animals think and feel just as we do. When I communicate with animals I find they speak so openly and honestly. There's no guile.

If you truly want to communicate in this way, you need to be as present as they are. Being in a state of presence can be referred to as a meditative state. I used to envy how animals do this so naturally but am pleased now that I can achieve this for myself. I feel so in tune with them and myself now, more than ever before.

When meditation or focus comes easily, I call this getting into 'the zone'. This means any time I wish to be receptive to an animal, I merely have to slip into that quiet zone. My mind is then able to send and receive clear messages.

Remember, animals do understand what you say or think to them. Just for a day, every time you do anything—from driving the car to washing the dishes—try to be in the present. Don't allow your mind to drift from the job you are doing until finished. If you find yourself drifting, that's okay. Just bring it back to your activity and continue on. You may find this difficult at first, as humans very rarely stay in the now.

Meditation would have to be one of the most effective and pro-health practices we could possibly carry out. Without doubt, people who meditate daily are more focused, relaxed and less stressed. Plus the power of observation is greatly increased, while blood pressure may be lowered too. And get this, twenty minutes of meditation is said to be equivalent to two hours of sleep.

Another exercise you can try is to spot meditate. This can be done by doing a body check. Every couple of hours, become aware of your body, checking if it's relaxed. See if your muscles are tense or relaxed, if your shoulders are up around your ears or in their correct position. When I first tried this, I was amazed how many times I discovered that I needed to lower my shoulders. The skin and muscles of my face—particularly on my forehead—were tense. It's downright scary to know how churned up we can get over the course of an average day.

Spot meditation can be done in many ways. Just take the time on a daily basis to look at an object such as a flower in a vase or an ornament; it doesn't matter what it is. Just lightly gaze upon it for a minute or two, and while doing that, clear your mind of other thoughts.

After doing these exercises for a while you'll notice a distinct change in your calmness, perception and focus. And so will animals. Imagine if you could maintain that level of focus in everything you do. Each activity would be done with so much more precision as all of your senses would be concentrated in one area. We need to place more emphasis on *now*—as it gives us the power to shape the future.

This was how I began my journey into the depths of meditation that is now available to me. The spot meditations were spontaneous, and extremely easy to execute. From five-minute meditations, concentrating on my breath, I progressed to fifteen minutes. From there eventually to an hour, and more.

If you want to connect with animals, you must remain in the same zone for the duration of the conversation. When you practice meditation regularly and feel the serenity it provides, you will find you'll want to be in this zone for longer and longer. And here's even better news: eventually this state of being will be the norm for you, and the frantic, busy feeling that was once a permanent fixture in your life will come along much less often.

Meditation is practiced by a relatively small percentage of the population in modern civilizations—although in more recent times it has greatly increased in popularity. Especially in eastern cultures, it is practiced regularly and has been done so for centuries. They see the wonderful benefits it provides. The stream of connectedness will be so simultaneous that intuitive conversation will happen in an instant, whenever required, with animals and with all of nature. What a wonderful place to be!

3

Was I Crazy?

ONE OF MY FIRST ATTEMPTS AT COMMUNICATING WITH AN ANIMAL, one I didn't know, happened when I saw a man walking his Boxer dog. As we came towards each other I silently said 'Hello' to the dog. I then explained my name was Trisha and that I was trying to learn animal communication. I asked if he'd mind having a word with me? The dog looked up in amazement and inquired if I was talking to *him*. Yes, I was.

He certainly wasn't used to speaking with humans, and he told me that while this man talked to him, he never seemed to hear the dog's response; therefore he presumed people didn't know how to converse with dogs. He seemed quite a character and had a good sense of humour.

As I wasn't used to this type of communication, it was hard to know what to chat about, so I simply asked the Boxer if he was enjoying his walk. *Yes very much*, he replied, adding that he'd have liked to been able to stop and sniff around a bit more. It seems the man would always urge him to keep moving when he tried to stop. That was an interesting perspective, as when I walked my dogs in years past, I remember doing the same thing.

The Boxer explained that sniffing different smells was a dog's way of knowing what was going on in the area, and which animals have recently been in the vicinity. In the wild, this would be crucial to their survival for picking up the whereabouts of prey and predators. We humans like to chat to people to find out information—whether they are work colleagues, family members or an acquaintance. We read newspapers or watch the news on TV to tap into what's happening in the world. Sniffing and exploring the environment is a dog's way of discovering the same information.

A dog's life is usually within the confines of a house or backyard. If you think about it, you realise how important checking out the smell and territories of other animals is to your dog when out and about. Perhaps we all need to take more time to let them be a dog when we're out on a walk.

I was right at the beginning of a journey of discovery. Not only was I talking to animals, but was, at the same time, learning and understanding their ways. Being so eager, I couldn't wait for my next encounter.

On another occasion when I was taking a long walk around the bay, I spotted an unusual-looking bird. I decided to see if it would give me any information, so I asked what it ate. It showed me a mental picture of some sort of berries, and I thanked it. Then as I was walking away I wondered how could I prove to myself this actually happened. I always had an element of doubt and wondered if the information

I was receiving might have come from me, using what my logical mind put together and not from the animal.

When I reached the other side of the bay, I saw more of the same species of bird and, lo and behold, they were on the ground eating the berries I'd seen in my mind's eye. It doesn't always happen that way, but it was great validation on that occasion.

Excited by these early experiments, I wondered what I should do next. There was one sure way of getting routine feedback that I was on the right track—but I knew it would be quite daunting. I was nervous about asking people for permission to talk to their animals so I could then tell them what their animal said. I was concerned at what their response might be. I'll be honest with you: I was a little nervous at the prospect of being laughed out of town!

Even though I was scared, there was something in me that longed to be the voice of all animals. I decided it was worth the skepticism, but first I'd put my toe only in the shallow end by asking my own family to let me loose on their animals. Family loves you no matter what, and I hoped they'd believe that what I was ready to share with them was something genuine.

I was about to fly without a net. Here goes!

4

Contessa the Family Cat

CONTESSA IS MY FAMILY'S MUCH LOVED, PART-CHINCHILLA CAT.
She can appear standoffish, preferring her own space—but
we're all like that at times, aren't we? She doesn't need people
or other animals to make her life complete, and occasionally
I envy her that independence.

She enjoys a short play when it suits her, but tires easily
with boredom. Contessa's a very regal creature who definitely
has a mind of her own—and she'll make sure you know about
it. Preferring to be in a quiet area rather than where all the
commotion is, she spends most of her days in her special
enclosure under the trees in my mum's backyard.

Pete and I travelled to see my family for a few weeks over
Christmas and one day Mum and I peeked out the window
at Contessa who was sound asleep in her hammock. I called
her name silently several times, and suddenly she woke up
and looked around. Mum saw this happen, but pointed
out that Contessa may have simply woken because she'd
heard a noise—everyone's a critic! I realised then that I'd

have my work cut out winning over my family to animal communication! So I waited until Contessa was fast asleep once more, then called her silently again—and the same thing happened.

For Mum's benefit, I then told Contessa to look over towards the window. Her head started to turn, when suddenly I had an impulse to imagine I was looking through her eyes, allowing me to see what *she* saw as she turned towards the window. I did this, and sure enough, she turned and looked directly at us. My mother thought it was amazing. 'Yes it is,' I said. 'It's animal communication.'

Then something incredible happened in my own backyard, so to speak. Peter and I were in a rented apartment with Mattie and Shea. The owner had decided to sell the place, and Marjorie the agent began opening up the apartment to the public every weekend.

At first all four of us would go out for a couple of hours, then return when everything was finished. Majorie could see how disruptive this was, so she said we could leave Mattie and Shea there during the inspections. This seemed like a great idea as Mattie and Shea didn't like being taken away from home, and Pete and I could use the time to do our shopping.

Our babies became quite a drawcard to prospective buyers, and spent a lot of time with Marjorie over a few weeks. Mattie and Shea were even used in the photographs for the advertisement, which was truly cute. We were so proud of them. Then one day during the week, I came home in the afternoon and found a light on. I was positive I'd turned all the lights out before I had left. Instinctively, I knew somebody must have been in the apartment, so I immediately rang

Marjorie. She said she hadn't been there, as she knew she had to ask my permission first, and that I'd probably just left a light on by mistake.

I hung up then turned to Mattie and asked her if anyone had been in the apartment, and I immediately saw pictures of Marjorie and a man in work boots walking down the hall. I rang Peter and told him the whole story. But there wasn't much I *could* do apart from ringing Marjorie back and filling her in on what Mattie had said—but she didn't know that I could communicate with animals, and I didn't want her to think I was making it up to accuse her. So I decided to forget about it.

First thing the next day Marjorie rang, very apologetic. She said she'd been awake all night, upset because she'd lied to me. Turns out she had in fact gone into the apartment with a builder to take some measurements, as he happened to be in another apartment in the building when she called him, and he could to do ours then and there. It seems there wasn't time for her to phone me first.

So, trust me, next time you're alone with someone else's animals, be careful what you say or do, they may just tell their owner!

5

Shea and Mattie Show Me the Way

I BEGAN TO DO PRACTICE EXERCISES WITH MATTIE AND SHEA on a daily basis, and this enabled me to increase my skills and experiment with different ways of using this type of communication. I found it crucial in the early days to keep validating my results to gain confidence and to strengthen my belief in what I was doing.

Quite often I would silently call to Mattie or Shea when either one was in another part of the apartment. After my second try at it the one I called would casually walk into the bedroom as if to say, *Yes, did you want me?*

One day Mattie was lying on the floor beside my bed. I sent her a visualisation, showing her jumping onto the bed and coming to me. The image in my mind was as if I was watching those very actions from above.

It took a few attempts on my part before she jumped up onto the bed and came to me. She said, *Didn't you think I would come? I got your message, and it became clearer the more you tried.* I tell you, I almost jumped for joy.

Mind you, trying the same exercise with Shea was a totally different experience. Showing him the same visual actions didn't work. At first I couldn't understand why, because I'd repeated the message several times, as I'd done with Mattie. Then Shea looked up at me, stared into my eyes, and suddenly a different idea popped into my head—I honestly don't know, though, whether this was actually my idea or Shea's. I imagined going inside Shea's body and looking out through his eyes, just as I'd done with Contessa.

I began viewing my bed at *his* height in my mind, how it would appear to him and imagining what I'd look like, standing across the other side of the bed. It felt strange at first, but then I began seeing things from his perspective more clearly. Next thing Shea was up on the bed and walking toward me saying, *That's it, you got it, Mum.*

I realised then how important the sending of this information was. Depending on the animal and the circumstances, these messages may need to be sent in one of several ways. Let's face it, if a message isn't clear, how could I ever expect any animal to respond.

One night I asked Mattie to sleep on the pillow next to my head, which was something she'd never done before. I told her this would be a sign for me, validating my communication with her. She did as I asked for the next two nights, but then never slept there again. I asked Shea to do the same thing, and he too slept beside my head for two nights. I wondered why they did it for two nights, not just one. They said humans are so skeptical that once may have been seen as a coincidence. Two was more of a sign. They were so right, because I definitely would have been unconvinced if they'd only slept beside me once.

Many of these visualisation exercises took a lot of focus, so daily meditation sessions were a must for me. I was understanding very quickly that when I had a quiet mind this communication came easily. Initially my meditation was only for a few minutes a day, but gradually I was able to increase it to half an hour, and then an hour, and so on. I found it necessary to be disciplined, as it was so easy to let days go by without any meditative practice.

There are many other things, such as our jobs, families and day-to-day activities, that occupy our time, and it can be difficult finding time for ourselves. If you see meditation as a priority, you'll make room for it, no matter how busy you are. Mastering this intuitive communication was important to me so I had to find time or I wouldn't improve. It was up to me.

Whenever I meditated, Mattie lay on my lap to somehow balance and calm me. Shea began to sit in on the meditations too, and this made it easier. I relied on them so much in those early days. Mattie became my teacher and helped me move along consistently in my development. Mind you, if I asked her to do the same thing too often, she'd remind me I was past that stage and didn't need any further validation. She was a hard task master, and seemed to be enjoying this authority a little too much. We all know people like that, but in the case of Mattie, her fundamental sweetness made her bossiness easy to forgive.

Mattie soon became known as 'Queen' around the house as she tended to preside over us all. Although she could at times get moody and impatient, she was extremely loving, affectionate and tolerant when it counted. She also had the ability to be the silent observer—all knowing and all seeing. Disturbances, such as raised voices or turbulent activity, caused her great distress, and usually she growled if they persisted. I felt she was telling us to not do it, or to get over it! She was indeed a cat who needed peace and harmony. We shared great communication together, and I loved the way she'd answer my spoken words with her verbal feline tones. It was as if it was Mattie's way of saying she could speak any language, including mine. She was definitely my best friend and mentor. Although amazingly intelligent and mature she was every bit the girlie girl, enjoying her bling nametag, and strutting as she walked.

Shea, on the other hand, was the strong, silent type. You'd never hear him approach, but he was always there. He enjoyed physical contact so much that he'd cuddle up in the crook of your arm whenever you were sleeping, or lie down beside you at any time of the day. He liked to take his time getting into an exact position—even if it meant I'd have to rearrange myself to accommodate him. Shea was very slow and deliberate in his movements and gestures, often reminding me of a lion. He tended to be playful for a while, and then he'd tire of the game. Interestingly, while Shea needed a variety of things to keep him amused, he often preferred a more laid-back approach to life—so he was kind of two personalities in one.

Shea was my complex cat, and like Mattie, could be a real bossy boots. He'd become quite loud when he'd decide to be vocal, as though some need of his wasn't being met. If I acknowledged him vocally, he'd suddenly slip into a relaxed mode, or maybe appear quite shocked that I'd heard his protest. I loved having him around me, as he was so calming, seeming to take all my stress from me. He was so much my beautiful handsome boy.

As I was getting more confident about communicating with animals, it was time to branch out and approach friends, colleagues and acquaintances to see what I could pick up from *their* animals. People took a while to come to grips with what they thought was just a hobby of mine, so there were mixed reactions to my offers to work with their animals. But most were positive. 'Mrs Dolittle' became a common nickname for me, but that was to be expected and, actually, I rather liked it.

Those who knew me well didn't need a lot of convincing; the rest, once I communicated with their animals and gave them information I couldn't have otherwise possibly known, began to change their minds. People began pursuing me to talk to their animal companions.

I was off and running towards an unusual and wildly rewarding career!

6

Tally: The Horse that Wanted to Leave

IT WAS STILL EARLY DAYS IN MY NEW ADVENTURE, SO I CONTINUED on with my career in dentistry as I learnt more about animals. One day Gina, a dental colleague and avid animal lover, told me about an animal communication workshop in a town several hours away. Of course I enrolled instantly, and Gina decided to join me.

We travelled down on a Friday night and the drive was mostly through a rural setting with many farms. Honestly, though, I really didn't care about the view, because all the way there I was becoming more and more excited about what lay ahead that weekend. We arrived late in the night at a small, quaint country town with just a few shops—mostly arts and crafts—along with one hotel, two restaurants, a small supermarket and a post office. There was only the one motel, just around the corner from the main road, and my first impression of the area was how chilly it was, compared with the city.

Really, it could have been at the edge of a cliff for all I cared. The only thing that mattered to me was this amazing opportunity. I was on the brink of learning more about talking to animals and was delirious with joy at having the chance to further develop this wondrous skill. It was hard to get to sleep that night, and after napping for only a couple of hours, I woke very early and readied myself.

We set off to find the property where the workshop was to be held, as it was on the outskirts of town. After making a few wrong turns we finally arrived at the farm, and as we drove up the long driveway, our anticipation escalated.

There were a lot of horses as we neared the house. Suddenly, at least six dogs appeared and came running out to meet us. We were welcomed by Julia, the animal communicator, and her husband, John. They showed us inside the farmhouse where we met the other participants, and of course they took us around to formally introduce us to all the animals around their property.

After we had sat by the fire with a cup of tea and become fully acquainted with everyone, we felt ready to begin. Unfortunately one of Julia's horses, Tully, her special friend, was gravely ill and she needed to wait for the arrival of her regular vet. She explained that Tully was a gentle, quiet being who had always been her inner strength and assisted her in her work, especially when it involved rescuing injured or unwanted animals. His illness had persisted over several months and quite simply was proving to be too much for Julia.

So on the day the workshop began, Julia's attendance was delayed, with John set to start us off with the initial exercises. There were six participants at the workshop, and we sat in the living area with notepads open and pens poised. John looked quite apprehensive and, although wonderfully friendly, was obviously not the usual teacher of these classes. He was, therefore, out of his comfort zone but he did his best.

Finally Julia came into the class and said the vet had arrived, and that perhaps we'd all like to witness the treatment. We gathered around Julia, Tully and the vet, Theresa, who began her examination, sharing her diagnosis with a deeply concerned Julia. This poor horse had a huge abscess on the side of his neck, which Julia had been draining. As I stood directly in front of Tully, he lifted his head to look my way and told me he wanted to go. I heard him clearly, and I was stunned.

At that moment Gina ran over, telling me she saw Tully look right at me. She asked me if he'd communicated anything, and of course I told her what he'd said. She then asked if I intended telling Julia—but looking over to Julia I saw how drawn and upset she was, so I whispered to Gina: 'I'm only the student and she's the teacher. I'm sure Julia will talk to Tully herself.' Gina then pointed out that maybe Julia was too upset to receive the communication clearly, and that perhaps Tully was relying on me to get the message across to his beloved owner. 'Think about it,' Gina continued. 'Why was he saying this to you and not to Julia?'

You can guess how nervous I felt. What if I had imagined the whole thing? But Gina convinced me I needed to approach Julia, so I moved closer to her and asked if she'd spoken to Tully. 'Yes,' she said, 'and he wants to stay. He wants to fight on.' With that, Julia moved away from us and back to be with Tully.

This of course was a great test for me and my belief. I knew what I heard was very clear, and I had in my mind that

Julia had told the class earlier, when we were sitting around the fire, that when your own animal is sick and you're very upset, it's more difficult to be objective.

An hour or so had passed and when Julia returned briefly to our group, I asked again how Tully was feeling. She said the vet's negative talk must have depressed Tully, for now he was saying he wanted to leave. At last Julia had heard what he needed her to know.

At the end of the day, when we were about to head back to our various motels that were scattered around the district, Julia asked if we could all go out to Tully and offer healing and support. It was starting to get dark and I felt compelled to crouch in front of him for more conversation. I silently asked how he was feeling. Tully said he was weary and didn't know how much longer he could hang on. I then asked, 'Why hang on? If you feel it's time to go—then feel free to leave.'

Tully knew his time was near, but didn't want to desert Julia if she needed him. I was now learning that this kind of death-bed dilemma occurs in the animal kingdom, just as it does in the human world. I felt sad, of course, but it was also incredibly exhilarating to have this revealed to me.

I could tell that his heart was heavy from watching Julia's torment and grief, and Tully knew once he was gone, the grief would continue. As he'd been her rock and companion for so long, it would obviously be hard for Julia to imagine life without him. I assured Tully that with Julia's abilities in animal communication, this would enable him to connect with her at any time. He could therefore assist her through her grief. I told him not worry, but to feel free to lie down and peacefully pass to the other side. There he'd be free of this terrible illness.

I suddenly felt so knowledgeable about the afterlife and what would occur, as if ancient wisdom had returned to my memory. It was one of the most profound moments of my life to that point. I sensed, immediately and powerfully, the interconnection between all creatures, and I understood that universal knowledge is available to each and every one of us once we're ready to receive it.

Gina and I then returned to our motel in a somewhat sombre mood, and after a brief dinner, we headed to bed after our very long day. The next morning I was awakened by a phone call from Julia's husband. He said that the workshop had been cancelled as Tully's condition had worsened. I felt compelled to ask if Tully was lying on his side and John replied, 'Yes,' sounding puzzled. 'As a matter of fact he is.' I thanked him for the call and told him our thoughts would be with them both. I knew now that Tully's time to leave was not far away.

Gina and I packed up with heavy hearts and headed back to the city. Travelling through the rural countryside, with Gina driving, I felt compelled to give her a running commentary on what animals I could see, and it wasn't long before there was a definite pause in my voice, and my eyes peeled to the left, taking in one particular paddock. In a quiet voice I said, 'Tully has passed over.'

Gina replied, 'What do you mean? How do you know?' Still with my eyes peeled to the paddock, I told her: 'I know because he's right there, running across the paddock, and he's transparent.'

Gina brought the car to a grinding halt, which really wasn't unusual for Gina. She immediately began to stare where I was looking. She said, 'All I can see is a paddock. I wish I could see him!' After a few minutes we continued on our trip, with me feeling I'd just taken another big step along my spiritual journey. And it all felt so natural.

That wasn't the last time I heard from Tully. Two days later I was driving home one night and an overwhelming feeling of love and warmth overtook my body. I asked in my mind whose presence I was experiencing. Then in my mind's eye a vision of Tully's face appeared. He was such a gracious loving being. I greeted Tully and he said he had come to thank me for my assistance that day. I told him he was very welcome and that it'd been a pleasure to meet him. With that, his vision faded and his presence was gone.

The experience with Tully was such a milestone for me. Over two days, I'd received clear, validated communication, forged great belief in my abilities, seen an animal spirit, and communicated with a deceased animal. What a mind-blowing weekend.

7

What the Geese Taught Me

I WAS SO FIRED UP AFTER THAT LIFE-ALTERING TRIP TO THE country, I decided it was time to refine my abilities and become a true professional in this strange and wonderful field of animal communication. This was definitely 'flying without a net' stuff for me, but somehow I wasn't nervous. I simply focused on my need to learn and experience as much as possible from the best teachers in the business—so I travelled to the United States where many renowned animal communicators conduct these intuition-enhancing courses. My time in America was to reinforce my conviction about how connected I already was to the natural world.

It was wonderful to be surrounded by like-minded people at the workshops, openly discussing our varied experiences. These people came from all walks of life, and were drawn so strongly to the animal kingdom and to nature in general. In other words, they were my kind of people and I was to make invaluable and long-lasting friendships there.

On that unforgettable trip, I went to a particularly special workshop on a farm in Oregon. And I have to say I was blown away by what a beautiful part of the country Oregon was—and I'm sure the heavenly surroundings helped in my quest. I was staying in town in Jacksonville, at one of those quaint southern-style B&Bs, with a four-poster bed and rose wallpaper. Luckily for me, Sharon, another person attending the same workshop, was also booked in there. She offered to drive me to and from the course, which was the kind of hospitality and generosity I discovered to be the norm in that neck of the woods.

The views driving up to the farm were breathtaking, and then suddenly before us was the quaint farmhouse surrounded on all sides by charming verandahs. I remember sitting there on one of the verandahs one day, scanning the full expanse of this fine property and sighing at the beauty of all I surveyed. It was at the base of glorious mountains and nestled in a valley. In every direction were steep inclines of pine forests. Paddocks were scattered in an orderly fashion across the landscape and were divided by timber fencing.

The animals ranged from dogs and parrots to sheep and llamas. There seemed to be a contented serenity across this farm—a scene completed by the sight of graceful humming birds hovering about. What a perfect place to be learning to achieve the inner silence and harmony needed to hear the words of the animals. It was a time in my life when I felt I had genuinely found paradise, and in that moment I knew in my heart that I was definitely on the right path.

The workshop began and, although we were all very enthusiastic, we were also a little bit apprehensive. Who wouldn't be? One of the exercises we were asked to do was to have a conversation with an animal we either feared, or felt was not particularly attractive to us. This was to help break down any barriers in the way we perceived certain animals; the fundamental background to this being that if our views were too fixed, this could prevent us from learning and experiencing that animal fully.

As I looked around, my eyes fell on the geese. Don't get me wrong: it's not as if I find geese unattractive, but out of all the creatures on this farm, they didn't particularly stand out to me. They didn't appear as interesting as the llamas or as enticing as the beautiful white fluffy Maremma dogs. So I chose the geese for my experiment. I then got straight down to business and asked them why they honked and made so much noise all the time. Instantly, one of the male geese—the largest of the group—came forward. He was a confident character, and it was clear why he'd stepped forward to respond, sending me a visual picture of all the students, myself included, having lunch earlier on the verandah. He showed our endless chatter, passing food and drinks, laughing and the like. He asked if I thought their species made more noise than my species. I had to admit he did have a point. He had me there, and I couldn't help giggling.

This big daddy goose went on to say that the honking sound they make was to alert other animals to strangers on the farm—both animals and humans. And more importantly, as he silently explained to me, the presence of the geese actually helped to unite all the animals. He described how they were the voice of the farm and its animals, all of whom relied upon their warnings and their communication to alert them to what was going on across the hills and dales.

You see, the geese were not confined to a paddock or yard, as were many of the other animals, but rather, they were free to wander to any area. Most people tended to ignore them as I had, so this made it easier for them to go unnoticed, the clever creatures that they are.

I was amazed at how much they understood what was going on around them. I discovered them to be extremely intelligent and confident, and with their funny webbed feet, they managed to waddle their way around the full extent of the farm several times a day. They reminded me of a group of girls on a night out, gossping, laughing and enjoying endless chick chatter.

8

A Delicate Balance

HAVING HAD MY CONCEPTIONS OF GEESE BLOWN OUT OF THE water, I got to thinking that the popular perceptions of many animals would change if this silent communication took place on a wider scale. We humans have a tendency to be preoccupied with our own ways of doing things, often making judgements about what's going on with the animals we know based purely on our limited outlook. Many of us see animals as having lower intelligence and significance. This just isn't so.

Our beliefs are often based on how closely another species resembles us and our behaviour. When you start to really communicate with them it enlightens you: you learn other ways of looking at things. Animal lovers know it's quite false to rate the value of animals according to their lack of a superficial resemblance to us.

There are stacks of differences between the species, from their genetics to their physical capabilities. The aerodynamics of birds and their ease of movement over long distances have assisted us in developing aircraft. I'm awed whenever I think about how birds were navigating with extreme precision long before we even took to the air. And I love it that people have come up with designs based on the sophisticated physical attributes of animals.

Just because animals can't write or operate a computer it doesn't mean they're less intelligent. The same applies to us. Who can fly to the heights of an eagle or swim to the depths of whales without mechanical assistance? Just because we can't do these things it doesn't make us physically useless. We may have bodily differences but that's no reflection on our mental abilities.

Speaking to the geese and the other animals that weekend made me realise every species needs to be honoured for what it is, and for its individual attributes. It's wrong to judge and put species into 'inferior' and 'superior' categories. Each of us has a vital place and role on this planet, and my personal mantra is, *we're all of equal significance.*

All animals must be given their space and importance. If we dominate them, we upset the delicate balance of life. We are, after all, just another species on this planet.

9

An Insect Moment

MY EARLY EXPERIENCES WERE NOT LIMITED TO FARM AND domestic animals. Guidance in my communication abilities tended to come from all areas of the animal kingdom. You can't imagine my surprise when a brown, flying insect talked to me one day. He had almost transparent wings and I hadn't seen anything like him before.

He told me right off that there was a slight restriction in my conversations with animals and that I needed to loosen up and ride like the wind, or float like a feather through the breeze. I realised he meant I was trying too hard, thereby forcing the situation. He explained I needed to sit back, relax and allow what's natural to occur. He went on to say my work with animals would become part of a bigger picture, and that nature would give me directions along this path. Furthermore, he said humans had a role to play in preserving this planet, and that together with the rest of the natural world we could all help change the earth's current environmental problems.

All this from an insect!

To say I was stunned is the understatement of the century, but it really did happen. Then came his big finish. When I asked him what I had to offer the world, he simply said that I could give back love, compassion and commitment.

I learnt that there are unlimited benefits for animals and humans to be able to communicate. Let's face it, without their ability to talk to us it's a very one-sided relationship. Now, thanks largely to a kitten, a goose, an amazing horse and a brown insect, my abilities had been honed sufficiently to take on the world.

PART II

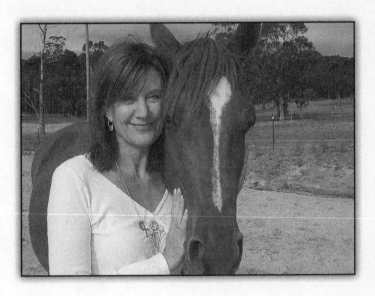

My New World

10

Melita: An Unhappy Horse

MY FIRST PAYING CLIENT WAS ROWENA. SHE WAS AS MEMORABLE as her horse, Melita, who had all the traits of pre-menstrual tension (and I'm talking about the horse here, not the human!). Boy, did Melita have a bad attitude. Rowena was at her wits' end with her horse's constant outbursts of appalling behaviour. Melita would be okay one day, then all of a sudden she'd become aggressive with Rowena and end up being completely unmanageable.

Rowena was hoping I could shed some light on the problem, as she'd got to the point of considering selling Melita, thinking the horse might be happier elsewhere. I had a gut feeling I could get somewhere with this tricky situation and, after a lengthy conversation with Melita, it appeared she may have been judged too harshly. Although she had quite a dominant personality, like so many animals we find difficult, her past was actually determining her present attitude.

It turned out the poor thing had been passed from home to home, and never felt nurtured by whoever she was with. Melita gave me quite a detailed description of her previous owners and, sadly, she hadn't been a special horse to anyone. She'd been kept in a very small stall, mostly in the dark, for many days, if not weeks, at a time. When she was ridden, the ill-fitting bit tore her mouth and, if she made a fuss, she was beaten. No wonder Melita had such a strong stubborn side, with a will to match. I soon discovered that she had great respect for who she was, and for her species, and wouldn't let go of that lightly. If provoked, she'd stand her ground, but could be fiercely loyal to the right person; however, that person was going to have to earn it.

I loved stripping away the layers of hurt that Melita wore like a suit of armour to find out more about the beautiful girl underneath. She was an animal that needed to have choices, and she required an environment that would give her a sense of internal and external freedom. In other words, she needed to have adjoining paddocks where she was free to roam from one to the other.

Being agisted in a small paddock with other horses not of her choosing, as she currently was, wasn't sitting well with her. Many of you will understand being bound restrictions and rules, like when you are at school or in a job you don't particularly like. We all know the feeling.

I saw that beneath Melita's stern exterior lay a deep, deep longing for kindness and support. Melita loved Rowena, but because of her past experiences she still had a general distrust of humans. She told me that every time she'd start to trust someone and get close to them, they'd sell her, and now even Rowena was thinking of getting rid of her.

I explained to Melita that if she curbed her behaviour, Rowena may decide to keep her. Melita, on the other hand, wanted to make it clear that her needs were important too, and they might not always fit in with Rowena's plans. She wanted to spend time with Rowena having fun, not always sticking to the routine. Melita explained that Rowena was far too serious and needed to learn how to have fun, but admitted that she wasn't sure why she always felt the need to punish Rowena with her challenging behaviour, because she did after all love her human very much.

We've all been stuck in that weird place of regularly hurting the one we love. It's a cliché, but it's one because it's true. I suppose it comes down to wanting to test the strength and durability of the relationship.

I suggested to Rowena that she give Melita another chance. I explained she should organise some sessions in natural horsemanship for boundary setting, and then put some time aside purely for play. As I saw it, Rowena needed to act to reinforce Melita's importance to her, incorporating mental pictures, and working on getting the message across that she wasn't going to sell her. I recommended Rowena visualise herself riding Melita out on a trail, or maybe doing some other activity they both enjoyed, and to picture them both having fun. This way she wouldn't have to choose words or explanations because, as we know, a picture paints a thousand words. This clear, yet simple, imagery would make it easy for Melita to understand what Rowena had in mind for their shared future.

Rowena then revealed to me that the information I'd uncovered regarding Melita's past was spot-on. She also told me she didn't really want to give her horse up and would try my suggestions. It certainly made things easier understanding what the problem was and how Melita was feeling. It's true in life that, no matter how well our intentions are, we never completely know the other side of the story unless we ask. To my delight, Rowena was happy to begin rebuilding their relationship. She had learnt that patience and understanding goes a long way.

When animals have been hurt or abused in some way, this sets them up to have trust issues and it can be traumatic for them if those memories resurface. Even though they may be in loving and nurturing environments with people who care for them deeply, it still takes time to rebuild trust and enthusiasm. Some never seem to fully move on and leave fear behind, preventing them from finding joy in new relationships. Sounds just like us, really.

11

Gerald the Pig

AS YOU GET TO KNOW YOUR ANIMALS YOU'LL FIND THAT EVEN small changes in their environment or conditions can have a great impact on their emotional and physical health. Like us, they have personal preferences that are extremely important to them, and if these aren't met they can become physically ill.

This is what happened to Gerald, a rather large very handsome pig who's one of the nicest pigs I know. I could hear the concern in the voice of Renee, who looks after Gerald, when she rang to say he'd become listless and depressed. It seemed he'd gone from being very energetic to an extremely lethargic boy.

I was quite surprised about this. When I'd first talked to Gerald he'd had this uncanny sense of humour. What a character! He reminded me of an elderly gent who carries a bit of weight, wears old-fashioned glasses and tells funny stories to whoever will listen. That was the Gerald I knew, so I was bewildered as to why this had suddenly changed.

I went to see Gerald and asked him what was going on. He said he was feeling down, as he used to be a lot closer to Renee. I told Gerald how Renee loved him. He said he knew that, but the problem was they used to spend more time together. He showed me in my mind's eye how Renee and he used to watch the nightly news on TV together. I saw them both sitting there, eating delicious doughnuts with jam centres and having enormous fun.

I thought I must have this wrong. Gerald sitting indoors, watching the news on TV and pigging out, so to speak, on junk food? He was a *farm* animal for goodness sake!

I needed to clarify this with Renee, and so I explained what Gerald had said. She told me they did used to watch the news together, with Gerald on the couch and her on the floor next to him. On occasions she'd bring out a plate of jam doughnuts—so the image I was getting from Gerald was accurate.

After replacing the couch twice, Renee felt that enough was enough, as her bank balance wouldn't allow her to keep buying new furniture. So she built Gerald a room close to the house, where she could see him and talk to him. But Renee had no idea that this thoughtfulness on her part was actually causing his unhappiness.

I went back to Gerald and explained that Renee was trying to spend as much time as possible with him, and the proof of this was that she had made sure his new room was close to the house.

This didn't cut any ice with my pig friend, who insisted he really missed watching the news with Renee: it had been their special time together and it had allowed him to be truly part of her human world, even if just for a short while.

I relayed this back to Renee. She was keen to have the old Gerald back so she immediately put a small television in his room and they began watching the news together again. She also brought doughnuts to share with him. Within days, Gerald was back to his old self. He even asked me on my next visit if Renee could also bring marshmallows to their evening get-togethers in front of the television. Being a very smart pig, he was trying to take advantage of this unique opportunity.

Gerald may have been a farm pig, but he wanted to keep abreast of what was going on in the world by watching the news, and if he could also wangle a few yummy treats out of Renee, then even better. It just goes to show we should never assume anything about any of God's creatures. More times than not they're way smarter than we think. Mind you, even though Renee has done her best to maintain a great connection with Gerald and consider his needs, there still must be some boundaries. This is why Gerald is still not allowed in the house and on her couch, but only on a soft mattress in a room off the house. Gerald is now one merry pig. How do I know? He told me so.

12

The Wisdom of Dogs

THERE'S A POPULAR EXPRESSION THAT GOES, 'YOU'RE EITHER a dog person or a cat person'. But plenty of us enjoy the wonderful attributes of both. As different as they are, cats and dogs offer a special and amazing experience when we fully let them into our world. I'd be hard-pressed to think of many people who haven't had one or the other living with them at some point, and I'm afraid I feel sorry for those who haven't had either. But in this chapter, let's consider what's wonderful about dogs.

What is it about a small puppy that melts your heart the moment your eyes meet? The longing to pick them up and squeeze them in your arms. Sigh! Dogs never hesitate in showing affection, and this makes us feel good about ourselves. It's heaven, isn't it, to come home after a hard day at work and there's your canine friend, waiting for you in a state of excitement that you've returned? I have often commented to my husband that I've never seen him act that happy when *I* arrive home!

On a daily basis, dogs show great appreciation for us in so many ways, and I feel this is a constant reminder to us to be more open with our feelings to those in our lives—whether animal or human. It's amazing how in a matter of moments a dog can totally change our mood, to one of laughter and joy through a funny antic, or by their constant display of warmth and attention. The love of a dog shows us how we should not only truly value ourselves, but others too. This helps us to keep in perspective what the truly significant things are in our lives, and not concern ourselves with the trivialities.

I love the way dogs play without the focus on who wins. In fact their lives revolve around fun. It doesn't matter what the game, or how it turns out, they just know how to get pleasure out of simple things. You won't find sore losers leaving a dog game, unless they are human, of course! Dogs are always honest in everything and every way they interact with us. We can always be sure of their truth and love.

Dogs rarely have bad days, and you know why? They're eternal optimists, and we can benefit from that. We're actually less likely to focus on fears and disappointments when we share our lives fully with a canine family member (or two). Dogs are never too busy to give us what we ache for. They don't have expectations, or need to question our motives. They just accept what we offer.

In *our* world, life can throw us many ups and downs. Whichever way it goes, your beloved puppy dog will be there to support and comfort you. It's the strength of this type of loyalty and commitment that keeps us moving forward in our lives.

When I was in my early twenties, my life was quite chaotic with a busy career and then my parents' divorcing.

The whole family was under a lot of strain. Some days it was just too much, and I'd go out the back of the house to shed some tears in private—alone, except for trusty Winston, my Maltese Terrier, who was always close by. He'd just sit there quietly beside me on the back steps, gazing into my face, occasionally giving my hand a slow, tender lick, as though to say: *It's okay Mum, I'll look after you.* His sweet little face soon stopped the tears and we'd hug for a while, and then chat. Miraculously, the dark clouds would lift from me, at least for a time.

I have no doubt that plenty of you have been comforted in this way by a dog friend. Winston became my rock in so many ways during those difficult times. You don't need to have a prominent career, a luxury car or a million-dollar house to be appreciated by a dog. They couldn't care less how much money you have or don't have in the bank, because they see far beyond such superficialities. They know what's important, and they can show us the way.

Darling creatures that they are, they love us for who we are right now. While we're taking care of our beloved dogs, they're constantly encouraging us to be strong and positive. As dogs have such simple attitudes, they teach us to take the clutter from our lives and fill it only with the things that matter. In a nutshell, they teach us to think positively about ourselves and the world around us.

Dogs start each and every new day looking forward to something, however small, and we could do well to adopt that lovely philosophy. For instance, it's unbelievable how much pleasure taking a simple walk with your dog can be. Stress seems to literally melt away. Without realising, you have found a wonderful way to exercise and get healthy.

Walks also encourage interaction with other people, which wouldn't normally occur, and how fabulous is that! For some reason, when you see a person approach you with a dog, they appear to be friendlier than they might otherwise, and this makes it easy to strike up a chat.

Dogs have a wonderful way of showing you that, whether you are playing or on your special walk together, life can be so much fun. Even if the route of the walk never varies, there are discoveries to be made. If you observe carefully, your canines will introduce you to jewels in your environment you wouldn't have noticed on your own. It's as though that tree, plant or twig wasn't there yesterday; or if you had seen it previously, you'll be shown a whole new way of looking at it today.

It takes our senses to an enhanced state of awareness, allowing us to appreciate things we wouldn't normally hear, smell or see. It's teaching us how much of life we miss if we don't allow ourselves to stop and smell the roses.

13

Carlos's Lucky Escape

CARLOS WAS A RICH BROWN-COLOURED KELPIE. THIS WONDERFUL breed is often used as sheepdogs. They're smart, hyperactive and easy to train. I just love them to bits and I like nothing more that watching them round up sheep. It's one of the most entertaining sights you'll ever see.

My encounter with Carlos, however, didn't take place in this sort of situation, but in an animal refuge. One of his attendants, Sarah, who cared for him deeply, was concerned he'd never find a good home. Carlos had been with them for several months and in that time had built up a strong relationship with Sarah. It was strange, because Carlos was aggressive towards every other person he encountered, including the other staff members—everyone except Sarah. This behaviour seemed to be confined only to humans, as he got on beautifully with all the other dogs at the centre. Sadly his feral attitude meant the attendants didn't hold out much hope of ever finding Carlos a home. So it was looking as though he'd either spend the rest of his life in a small enclosure in a refuge or be euthanised.

Carlos had been found, lying on the side of a country road with a broken leg, by an elderly couple. He was very thin from lack of food, flea-ridden and full of worms. The couple were on their way back to the city when they saw him struggling to get to his feet, and the sight of this wretched creature was so utterly heartbreaking, they pulled over to assist him.

Poor Carlos was too weak to react to them, so they were able to lift him onto the back seat of the car. Unable to bear the thought of him being put down, they took off to find the nearest vet and gladly agreed to pay to have his broken leg fixed. Despite being animal lovers, they couldn't take on a dog as they lived in an apartment. That's how this poor dog ended up at an animal refuge.

Sarah would have happily taken Carlos but she already had several other rescued animals living with her and she was mindful she'd already reached her canine limit. Taking on Carlos as well was out of the question, much as she loved him. Contacting me was her last hope. No pressure of course!

When I got there, the first thing I noticed was that Carlos had the most sorrowful eyes. I instantly felt his inner pain. I just knew I had to unearth the sad events that brought him to this emotional scrapheap. He trusted me and I was soon hearing how he had lived on a farm with many animals, including three other dogs. He said the only friends he had in the world were these dogs, and the four of them used to round up sheep and cattle all day. But they were fed very little and were locked up in a metal shed when they weren't working. Carlos and the other dogs were punished all the time by the very big man who lived there. *We were either confined, or often beaten with wood,* he said. *We were not sure why. I guess we were bad or had made mistakes.*

Turns out, one day when Carlos was working hard at rounding up sheep the man began yelling at him. He picked up a piece of wood and hit the poor Kelpie on the leg, causing dreadful pain. Carlos couldn't get up, much as he wanted to, and the nasty boss kept threatening to hit him again.

At this point in the story Carlos seemed relieved to finally have the opportunity to let out all his sadness and rage, and I encouraged him to keep going, not that he needed much encouragement. After feeling isolated and wounded for so long, Carlos found his tale just came tumbling out. The man had become really angry when he saw that Carlos genuinely couldn't stand up, and was therefore of no more use to him.

I had tears streaming down my face as Carlos told me how he was so afraid, and that all he could do was cower into a small ball. Can you imagine Carlos's terror when the man chased away the other dogs who had come to see what had happened, and then threw him into the back of his vehicle? They drove for what seemed such a long time and then Carlos was unceremoniously dumped on the side of the road. He said he was in so much pain, and even though he tried many times, he couldn't get up. He didn't know how long he had lain there before the kindly couple came along, but it seemed like forever because he was so hungry and the nights were so cold.

Well, you didn't need to be a rocket scientist to work out why Carlos was so aggressive towards humans.

I asked Carlos what struck me as the obvious question: did he dislike people so much that he actually wanted to hurt them? *Oh no,* he said, *I just do that so they keep their distance, because I'm so scared of what people might do to me.*

Such a sensitive soul. His recovery from this terrible situation was going to be slow, due to his delicate state. Carlos had previously taken any punishment or harsh treatment personally, and now felt he had to be aggressive keep everything and everybody at a distance in order to survive. I asked why he didn't act this way to Sarah, and he said her kindness allowed him to trust her. Her, and no-one else.

I told Sarah his story and she broke down in tears and couldn't believe anyone would want to mistreat a beautiful creature such as Carlos. We both knew Carlos was deeply scarred, but in time things would improve. I was sure of that.

I suggested that the first steps may be to spend time with Carlos having fun, playing with a ball or taking him for a walk around the grounds. He needed to know that life could be joyful, and that being with people could be enjoyable and non-threatening. I also thought that inviting one of the other attendants along for a couple of these sessions would allow Carlos to get used to someone else being involved in these relaxed encounters. The other attendant could keep their distance at first, and over time get closer and closer, until actually being involved in the activity.

I stressed that these sessions had to end with Carlos being praised and being given his favourite treats, thereby creating a positive feeling for him about playing and interacting with people. In time, hopefully, he'd be happy to share his life with a new family. Sarah agreed, saying she'd keep me updated.

Several weeks later she contacted me, excitedly telling me how much he'd improved. Carlos was now accepting another person at the refuge, and the three of them had played many games together. He was showing signs of confidence around people, rather than venting aggression. You can imagine how pleased I was to hear that Carlos was liking his life for the very first time. I cried tears of happiness when I heard it.

Silent communication works extremely well in these situations, as animals don't find it threatening or imposing. In fact many animals have said to me they prefer this type of communication more than verbal talk, especially when they've never met a person before. I can understand this, as often there are times when *I* prefer it that way too—the big advantage of it being that you don't have your personal space invaded, and you aren't confronted with potentially intimidating body language.

Thanks to Carlos, and not for the first time, I was seeing that what unites humans with animals is far greater than what divides us.

14

Animals Deserve Respect

WITHOUT MEANING TO, WE CAN HURT ANIMALS WITH OUR attitudes and behaviour. It's easy to forget we have the power in the relationship, because they have to live in our world. Even things like the difference between their size and ours impacts on whether or not they feel happy or scared.

Imagine being a tiny Chihuahua looking up the legs and body of a tall person, all the way up to a scowling face. Then add to that, the scariness of having that person raise their voice at you. Think about it. This kind of thing must be extremely daunting for animals, especially given they can't tell you how overwhelmed they feel.

Remember back, if you can, to what it was like being a small child, when you'd done something you shouldn't have and your mother or father was upset and scolding you. Pretty frightening, when you're only little, because everything appears so much bigger and intimidating when you're very close to the ground. Then when we become adults we are more eye-to-eye to the situations and, hopefully less likely to be paralysed with powerlessness. We feel more confident about having our say and expressing our viewpoint. But Chihuahuas remain small into adulthood, so this particular outlook is permanent for them and I've often seen them shaking with anxiety, as no doubt you have too, which is a pitiful sight.

We need to remember that animals, like us, grow up and mature, and when that happens they should command the same respect as we humans expect for ourselves. It must be humiliating at times for an adult animal to be treated as a juvenile. Perhaps that's why certain unfavourable behaviours continue all their lives.

Gary, a single guy in his thirties, shared his life with Gunther, a nine-year-old Staffordshire Terrier. Gunther had been with him since he was a puppy and they'd shared many an adventure together. They were an appealing duo wherever they went, due in part to how friendly Gunther was to people of all ages, and to any other dog he encountered on his travels.

I was brought into the frame because Gary became concerned about Gunther's occasional aggressiveness to his small nieces and nephews when they visited, which was unheard of for this loveable Staffi. Being a caring uncle, Gary was worried that the children could be unintentionally harmed.

I sat down with Gunther and explained Gary's concerns to him. He was shocked at the suggestion he might hurt the little ones. I did my best to pacify him, explaining that his actions of late were behind Gary's nervousness, because he regards his nieces and nephews as very precious. Gunther did understand what I was telling him, and then he asked me to tell Gary what was going on.

Gunther said he was getting older, and he couldn't take it any more the way the children teased him, however playfully, as sometimes they accidentally stepped on his tail or fell on his legs, which for a dog beginning to feel the effects of arthritis was truly awful. His response was always to hurriedly get out of the way to avoid considerable pain. Unfortunately he was now being branded as cranky by them. Gunther wanted me to make them aware of this and how he was older and needed his space to be respected. Yes, he was still happy to play, but with consideration given for his creaky bones.

Gary was relieved to hear that his pal was just getting older and hadn't lost his gentle, loving personality. He could now explain to his family what Gunther required at this time in his life, and that he needed to have his changed circumstances respected. He was sure the children would understand and be able to experience and enjoy Gunther's friendly nature once more.

The feedback I received later was that this is exactly what happened.

Sometimes the physical appearance of an animal can easily detract from how their maturity and intelligence are perceived in the human world. They appear so cute, that it's easy to overlook the fact that they have emotional and spiritual needs that should be addressed. Some animals don't appreciate wearing multicoloured clothes with a hood complete with fabric ears! And the same goes for being carted around in designer carry bags or strollers. They may find this demeaning or embarrassing, even if the intention is honourable. There are other animals, however, that quite enjoy sharing these fun things with you, but they do need to be given the choice. Take Raz, a golden Silky Terrier who'd been rescued from the pound by Heidi, who was only twenty at the time.

Heidi felt an immediate strong connection when she saw dear little Raz. In just a few months they had forged a wonderful relationship. Heidi felt Raz was like a younger sister, such was the bond between them. So what was the problem that brought me into the picture?

Heidi wanted to make sure Raz was happy with her new life, and to find out whether there was anything more she could do. I already felt Heidi was understanding Raz exceptionally well, and this was confirmed when I began talking to Raz. She let me know she was content with her life and with Heidi. In fact things couldn't get much better. Raz had everything she wanted, so this was one satisfied Silky Terrier. The next part of our conversation I thought was priceless.

Raz told me that Heidi brushed her hair every day, lovingly adorning her with pretty ribbons. Raz not only thrived on the attention, but also the fact that Heidi wore the same coloured ribbons in her hair. Raz truly felt like Heidi's sister!

The important thing to remember here is that animals have thoughts and feelings just like you do. You wouldn't want your likes and dislikes ignored, and animals feel the same way. Whenever you're making a decision for an animal, take the time to consider what effect this will have on them. Some of our decisions can have a dramatic impact, for better or for worse, and for the lucky ones, like Raz, these decisions enhance their lives.

15

One of the Pack

DOGS ARE COMPANION ANIMALS. THEY ARE NOT MEANT TO BE alone—it's not in their nature. To be happy they need to belong to a pack of dogs. Where this isn't possible they look for this crucial sense of belonging elsewhere. If they're the only dog in the household they will definitely make you part of *their* pack.

Even if you have more than one dog, you'll still be part of that pack, and believe it or not, you'll determine how far up the hierarchy you sit by your attitude. My husband thinks he sits at number six, which is the bottom of the hierarchy at our place. He could be right.

I'll never forget meeting Morris, a small, feisty Jack Russell who was driving Kirsty and Adam mad. They'd come home after working all day to find several large holes dug in their garden. The dirt would be scattered all over the patio, as would some of the plants, not to mention the lawn. Adam would scold Morris, then spend the next hour cleaning up the backyard. They'd spent a fortune on replacing many of the plants that didn't survive.

Let me say here that it's important to know that if you scold an animal, it needs to be done at the time of the incident, otherwise they don't have the faintest idea why you're annoyed. After several weeks of frustration Kirsty and Adam contacted me to see if they could get to the bottom of the problem. It was a clear-cut case of boredom.

Morris had energy to burn and needed to expend it somewhere. Morris also told me he was frustrated, as he was rarely taken for walks or a good run down at the park. And he mentioned that a playmate would be good too. Morris clearly had to have more activities to keep him occupied during those long hours alone. He also needed a lot more attention from Kirsty and Adam.

I passed all this information onto them, suggesting that an early morning walk before they left for work would make a difference. I recommended more toys for Morris and other things to amuse him in the yard. Perhaps, too, they could arrange for a dog walker to come during the day. I also mentioned the idea of a playmate for Morris, which at first wasn't met with a lot of enthusiasm, but Adam said he'd consider it.

As dogs are often confined to a backyard or inside a house, they must be walked regularly. If possible, they should be walked daily and, where permitted, allowed off-lead in an open space to run and explore in the unique way dogs have of ferreting around. They need to have freedom, just as we do, to make decisions for themselves. They love to run and chase balls, and look at different things. If you have more than one dog you'll see them play together for hours on end, just as children do. This is great stimulation and exercise for them, and the result will be much happier, healthier dogs.

Just for a minute, close your eyes and pretend you're a dog. Try to imagine what it feels like being on your own for hours with nothing to do. If it were practical, it would be good for us all to just sit in the backyard for eight hours without any diversions and see what it would be like. If all you saw was the back of a house and the fence, you'd go stir-crazy within the first sixty minutes.

Imagine hearing strange noises you didn't understand. Of course you'd bark to ward them off. Or you might hear another dog bark in the distance, so you'd bark back to let them know that this was your territory, or maybe you'd just want to talk to them. You're lonely as you wait with eager anticipation for someone to come home to either let you in, or at least interact with you. As a human, would you be happy with that life? If not, think about why not.

Boredom and anxiety can build erratic and unwanted behaviours in your canine friends. I'm sure I don't need to tell you—especially those of you who have dogs—just what a bored dog means! For starters, you're likely to end up with those endless holes in the lawn or garden, and ruined pots and plants, washing ripped off the line, ripped flyscreen on your doors, chewed lounges . . . the list goes on.

It really helps to make up new games for them, to hide food in spots around the yard, especially if you know you're going out. This will keep them amused for hours. Oh, and make sure they have plenty of toys. These are easy tasks to do, and you'll be rewarded tenfold.

Animals have just as much right to happiness as we do. They go to great lengths to fit into our world, and we should recognise and understand *their* world, whatever species they may be. We certainly expect them to understand *our* domain when it comes to rules and regulations, and it's important to remember that every relationship is built on give and take.

We're extremely fortunate with animals, as it's the simple things we do that create the greatest happiness for them—whether it is spending time stroking your feline companion, or a quick game of fetch the ball with your active canines. Why not make them as happy as they make us? I assure you that you'll be pleasantly surprised at the difference it will make in your life—the rewards are immense.

Go for it!

16

Habits that Drive You Crazy

EVEN THE MOST ARDENT ANIMAL LOVERS CAN BE SORELY TESTED: dogs barking excessively, digging holes in the backyard, chewing your precious belongings, wrecking the flyscreen door, or leaving toys everywhere; equally, cats dropping fur, scratching and peeing on the furniture, and male cats spraying. These irritations, however, are no worse than being bugged by a partner leaving the toilet seat up or down, and leaving clothes and belongings everywhere. Or screaming children leaving toys all over the floor and muddy footprints on the carpet. They're part of life, and they won't kill us.

While some people's bad tendencies are capable of being shed, it is often more difficult for an animal to make changes when their behaviour is caused in some way by humans. We need to understand what's going on, and look at ways to modify what's happening to solve problems.

Dogs bark partially because of genetics and partially through domestication. Barking is a form of communication. Dogs have descended from wolves that bark or howl when necessary. Humans developed the dog out of the wolf and encouraged barking so these animals could be used as watchdogs. The encouragement to bark actually started with people.

Wolves are never alone throughout their lives because they move in packs. When we bring dogs into our families, we're basically replacing their natural pack structure with our own. It's therefore not surprising that a dog left alone all day will bark consistently. In the wild, wolves would only bark in certain situations, and communicate silently with their pack in other circumstances. Domesticated dogs have to get their needs across somehow and, as most people don't use telepathy, barking is their only option.

Being bored can also contribute to the other so-called 'bad habits'. Dogs need company, activity and attention. It's part of their DNA. You can hardly blame them for acting on instinct. Perhaps that's why some dogs have been bred unable to bark—to fit in with the human way. I find this grotesque.

People spend hundreds of dollars on animal behaviourists, special anti-barking collars and sprays to curb a dog's barking tendencies. I would argue that telepathic communication is the first step in this process as you need to find out why a particular animal is behaving in this manner. The reasons for the conduct, however, are not always straightforward.

This was the case for Lisa, who had an adorable eighteen-month-old chocolate Labrador called Salvador. He was the only animal with Lisa and was left in the backyard during the day while she was at work. According to neighbours he barked incessantly. In desperation, Lisa tried collars, sprays and specialist companies specifically set-up to tackle barking. Nothing seemed to work. She came to me in the hope some questions would be answered and solutions found.

I liked Salvador instantly, sensing his serious nature. Although very loving and affectionate, the way he came across to me disturbed me slightly. He felt his job was to protect the family and his home. Every time he heard a noise, he'd bark furiously to keep any possible intruders away, letting them know not to enter—or else pay the consequences. Salvador felt that this barking warned both humans and animals that this was *his* territory. He wanted to contribute something worthy as he loved his home and Lisa very much. He insisted she was pleased with his efforts, and that he would never allow any harm to come to her.

So as you can see, darling Salvador was carrying a lot on his shoulders. When I explained this to Lisa, she was quite surprised because she'd presumed he was simply bored or overly sensitive to noise. Then, on giving it some thought, she realised she'd actually contributed to the problem.

When she'd first moved into her small house she was robbed within the first month, and this had made her nervous. She decided to get Salvador. He was only eight weeks old and quite hyperactive. Lisa was working part-time then, so he was inside with her much of the day, and when Lisa heard noises, inside or outside, she'd become anxious, which encouraged Salvador to react. So this was definitely a learnt behaviour on Salvador's part.

Now that she was working full-time, and not home for long hours during the day, Salvador was left outside, accessible to all sorts of different noises. Lisa felt guilty for yelling at him over his barking, as she could see that she was partially to blame. Lisa knew he was such a great companion for her; they had great fun and knew they'd be together a long time. Both of them told me they felt this strongly.

At my suggestion, Lisa, began the reprogramming. It took a lot of patience. She'd praise him when he barked at certain noises, and discourage the others. In time, his barking was greatly reduced and the neighbours were much happier. He became a calmer dog, now knowing, after some explanation from me, that his job was important, but that it didn't need to be carried out with such vigour.

Back to my previous comment about moderation in all things: the truth is that dogs do bark, but it's not right to scold them every time they do it . . . although there's no doubt boundaries are a must.

17

Being Present with Your Animals

I LOVE TO WALK MY JAPANESE SPITZ DOGS, AKEIRA AND SAVANNAH, each morning, usually in the forest near where we live. It gets me out of bed in the morning, and sets me up for the day. It's good for them and good for me.

Although the smaller in stature, Savannah, with her outgoing nature, streams out in front, leading the pack. She's an 'out there' dog, and very trusting; not afraid of anything unless it gives her reason to be. I should add that she's extremely inquisitive about everything, and overwhelmingly friendly to strangers of all species. So you can imagine the many stops and starts we make along the way as we pass various humans and their dogs. Any adventure is a good adventure for Savannah.

Akeira, on the other hand, can be anxious with new people and animals. She's also wary of unfamiliar places and situations—the opposite of her pal, Savannah. Extremely loyal, Akeira makes me feel important when we're out on our walks because she rarely leaves my side, as if to make sure I'm okay.

Chalk and cheese they are, and I love to watch their level of excitement escalate as they discover new smells and other creatures along the way. The forest is a mass of the most beautiful, ancient trees, making a wonderfully shaded canopy. The lower levels of plant life change dramatically as you move through it. It just shimmers. There's one area full of tree ferns that amazes me the most. You're completely surrounded by these lush green fronds for as far as the eye can see. You feel completely enveloped by living, breathing nature. The two dogs love running through this enchanted space, experiencing what we call 'The Land of Tree Ferns'.

There's another place we've dubbed 'The Magic Forest'. It's completely secluded, with a waterfall cascading down over large rocks, and then the water gently flows down to a small pool. The dogs and I enjoy sitting there, taking pleasure in its tranquility.

Being able to fully communicate with Akeira and Savannah makes the journey so much more interesting. They can tell me firsthand what they're seeing and how they're feeling. It's wonderful each day to be able to ask the dogs which part of the forest they wish to visit. You know, when I'm in the forest with Akeira and Savannah, it's as though the rest of the world doesn't exist. It's like we've actually created our own.

I have often thought of how animals make such an extraordinary contribution to our lives. Even our homes become richer for having their presence. A house begins as a dwelling to provide shelter and comfort, and once you add animals, it miraculously turns into a real home with warmth.

Take the animals away for one day and I swear it will turn back to being just a dwelling.

Sharing your life with a dog and observing their qualities makes us appreciate that they have traits *we* would love to possess. Living with them over time helps us to develop these desirable traits. I'm thinking in particular of strength, confidence, undying loyalty—and a great capacity for joy.

I love too that dogs have the uncanny knack of being able to get closer to us than most humans in our lives can. Our hearts feel safe and secure with our canine companions, and the incredible support they offer doesn't just impact on our emotional status, but also on our physical wellbeing. In a way, they can help us be the best we can be.

As talked about earlier, dogs form packs—with other dogs or with humans—and they love to interact within this pack, taking on different roles. They know how the pack functions at its best, and they can teach us great lessons about teamwork. I know for an absolute and divine fact that you will never be alone when you share your life with a canine—or with any animal for that matter. They are the ultimate in companions. Dogs and humans just seem to go together naturally and harmoniously, and it doesn't matter who you are or where you're from, you can share great happiness and understanding with a dog.

And if you give from the heart, that dog will reward you tenfold.

PART III

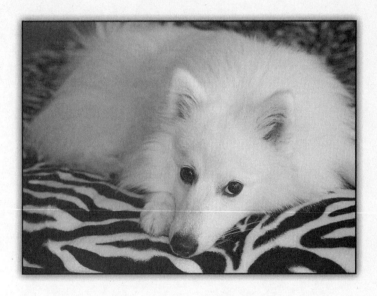

The Emotional Lives
of Animals

18

Sensing Illness or Injury

BEING ABLE TO INTUITIVELY CONNECT WITH ANIMALS HAS A great advantage when it comes to animal health. When you or I go to the doctor we're able to help with the diagnosis by telling the doctor any symptoms we're experiencing, but when we take an animal to the vet we often have limited information. We may know the obvious symptoms, such as vomiting, limping, or the fact they're no longer eating, but we don't necessarily know if they're in pain. Even if they're crying out, we're often unsure why.

If an animal is injured, then getting crucial information becomes even more urgent—it could save their life. Communicating with them and asking what they're experiencing is one way to get the facts. Are they in pain? Where is the pain? What else are they experiencing? The other way is by sensing or scanning their body intuitively to pick up the problem areas: that's called medical intuition.

When I began to develop this degree of sensing, I could feel the symptoms and sensations of my animals in my own body.

Think about it: when you communicate with someone who understands how you're feeling, it is a tremendous reassurance. I've had a number of ill animals tell me how much better they feel when they know I'm also experiencing their symptoms.

One of my first encounters with this type of sensation was when I visited Cynthia, a friend of mine. She owned a property a few hours from the city, which for me was like taking a breath of fresh air. Cynthia had an array of animals—horses, goats, pigs, dogs and chickens, even a stray peacock waiting patiently for a peahen to turn up to become his dream partner. Running down one side of the property was a beautiful forest of pine trees and native shrubs. To the other was a picturesque valley with a rambling stream. We're talking serious paradise!

After having a short chat and a cup of tea with Cynthia, I decided to go out to the paddock to visit her horses. As had happened so many times before, the horses came to say hello as I approached. One by one I greeted them by name and began chatting to them. I was instantly relaxed, as you would be when catching up with old friends.

Bob was the oldest in the group and obviously the leader of the pack. The other horses seemed to give him space, while Bob quietly observed the dynamics between the rest of them. Somehow he just seemed to have his finger on the pulse at all times. He was quite a guy, our Bob, and a standout for another reason: he was always reliable and consistent in every situation when it came to Cynthia. He was steadfast as far as she was concerned.

As I moved closer to Bob on this particular occasion he completely turned himself around, as if deciding to turn his back on me. This was unusual as he was normally very social and enjoyed a chat. My whole view of him was suddenly his rear end, which really wasn't quite what I had in mind! He then rested heavily on his back right leg, with his hips tilted.

As he had never done this before, I asked if everything was okay and, just as I did, I felt this agony in my left hip. I knew it wasn't *my* pain because it had come out of nowhere. I asked Bob if he was feeling discomfort in his left hip. He replied, *Yes,* and said that he'd been experiencing it for several days.

As soon as Bob acknowledged this, I no longer had the sensation of pain in my own hip. It vanished just as quickly as it had appeared. I was stunned.

I relayed this information to Cynthia and she realised that this must have been why Bob hadn't been keen to ride over the past couple of days. He wouldn't gallop and she was sure she had seen him limping on at least one occasion. Cynthia then organised treatment for Bob and he was relieved of his hip problem in no time. There are some great treatment options for horses—animal chiropractic, Bowen's therapy, and massage, which are some of the treatments that in my experience have proved a must for horses' health.

A word of warning here: even though medical intuition can assist, it shouldn't be seen as a diagnosis. It's only a tool that helps make the vet's or medical practitioner's job easier. As I have already mentioned, vets are sometimes working with limited information, and medical intuition can at times guide them to look in an area of the animal's body they wouldn't normally have considered. In Bob's case, it might not have been detected at all—or perhaps it might have been thought to be a foot or leg problem, which would have extended Bob's torture.

19

Natural Healing

ONE NIGHT WHILE I WAS CONDUCTING LIVE READINGS ON RADIO, Sally phoned in about her Schnauzer, Jack. She said he was a cheeky, fun-loving dog who rarely revealed a serious side. But this wasn't the case at the moment. He was extremely irritated and was scratching incessantly. Several vets suggested eliminating chemicals, changing shampoos and observing any excessive scratching around certain plants and grasses. Sally had to also fully monitor his diet, which she did. But nothing helped and, much to the desperation of everyone, a cause was never found.

After intuitively scanning Jack, I sensed his problem didn't have an external cause but an internal one. I suggested it might be cyclic, and involve an organ like his liver. He needed a blood test for more information to confirm what I was experiencing. So Sally took him back to her vet for tests, and the results were devastating.

Jack's enzyme count was anything but favourable. Follow-up tests with an ultrasound confirmed Jack had a liver issue and an impaired immune system. Usually by the time animals show the full symptoms of this disorder it's too late to help. The vets indicated to Sally that they usually see animals around eight to ten years old with this complaint, and by then the damage can't be reversed. At the very best you can expect a shortened lifespan and a lifetime on medication.

Vets have a very tough job, and it's wonderful if intuitive communication can assist this difficult work. Sally was extremely grateful as it had saved Jack's life. Due to early detection he needed medication only for the short term and is now back to the cheeky, playful and mischievous dog he had always been.

In my experience it's an advantage to get opinions from both conventional and wholistic vets. This enables you to look at your animal's health from many perspectives. Conventional and natural medicines can work very well together. In many cases, a natural approach is both very effective and all that is required, as animals respond well to nature's way.

Christie contacted me when her small Silky Terrier named Daisy was recovering from an operation to remove a tumour from the back of her eye. Daisy was seven years old and as sprightly as a puppy. To her, life was fun, fun, fun. She loved being involved in every single activity, large or small, with the family. This meant the human family, and the other three dogs. Christie was devastated that Daisy had also lost her eye and worried about the effect it would have on her. She wanted to know Daisy's feelings about the situation.

As soon as I began talking with Daisy her light, bubbly personality came through immediately. I asked her how she was feeling after the operation. She replied that it was no big deal. I sensed that her healing wound felt tight and sore and that the healing skin was dry and itchy. I reassured her that we'd place cream on her eye to take the itchiness away.

Daisy also agreed that seeing out of only one eye did feel strange, especially looking at certain angles. She went onto say she knew she was different now, but that it didn't matter as she could still run and play. She wanted me to tell Christie to stop worrying, because she'd be fine. She felt it was a bigger shock for Christie than it was for her. Daisy felt all this fussing, even though she did like attention, was getting a bit much. She didn't want her ailment continually brought up and talked about all the time. She just wanted everything to get back to normal, and not to be made to feel different.

Christie was so relieved to discover that Daisy was taking it so well, and was now confident of her recovery. She felt she could ease off on being over-sympathic now she knew that Daisy was eager for things to get back to normal.

There was another very similar case that still leaves me feeling goose bumps up my arms. Serena was a very sweet long-haired, tortoiseshell cat who had lost her tail due to a tumour. In the past she'd paraded around very proudly, making everyone aware of her beauty. Marina and Jacob, Serena's people, couldn't understand why every time they stroked her, she ran off. They were concerned she was suffering emotional scars from her tail removal.

When I communicated with Serena she was a little reluctant at first to discuss her medical issue, but I was patient and came to sense that when people stroked her, it felt like all the nerve endings were set off. She wanted me to ask Marina and Jacob to pat around her neck and shoulders instead. And she didn't want the loss of her tail to be a constant talking point. She was trying to get over the loss, and this was just a constant reminder. Serena insisted there was no guilt associated with their decision, as it wasn't anyone's fault. She just wanted things in the home to get back to normal.

I was deeply touched by the way Serena opened up and told me the reasons for her inner sadness about the loss of her tail. She felt that part of her was missing; part of her identity gone forever. I learnt from her that she used to have this really cute curl at the top of her tail which everyone commented on. She felt it was not only a very identifying part of her, but also a fundamental part of being a cat.

I felt tears on my cheeks as she admitted to feeling very embarrassed in front of the other cat, Sissy. She knew that the operation had to be done, but nevertheless it was hard for her. At that point I understood how support and encouragement would greatly help her. I wanted her to feel beautiful again and worked on convincing her that her coat was so distinct, and her eyes amazing; although she had lost her tail, everyone would now be able to admire her other assets. She said she hadn't thought of that.

Thank you gorgeous Serena for the lessons you taught me.

In the work I do, I'm not just treating an animal's physical injury, but all the facets that go hand-in-hand with that—their thoughts and emotions. There are many occasions where intuitive communication can also be used to help counsel an animal who's going through trauma—whether it is physical or emotional.

Many animals when afflicted with illness or injury just want to get on with their lives. They don't want to become a burden to their people, and they don't want their quality of life interrupted. Animals would prefer not to dwell on the negative of their situation but the positive. At times our stress and overanxiousness can make the circumstances worse.

Animals never cease to amaze me about how knowledgeable they can be. I was consulting a young dog, Athena, who had gone completely blind only a few months before. Most animals in this situation usually cope and adapt quite well. Athena, however, wasn't coping. She was bumping into things and becoming quite stressed. I asked her how we could help to make things a lot better for her. She immediately began to outline her specific needs.

Athena gave me the picture of door frames, and then the sense of the smell of lavender. It became clear she was asking for particular essential oils to be attached to door frames, and another smell for furniture, and perhaps another for steps. Introducing one smell at a time would enable her to recognise it, and what it meant, before introducing another. This way she could get about easily through her nose.

What an amazing dog to come up with this suggestion. I really felt I was being taught something that we humans could perhaps use to help blind people. Simple things that can make an amazing difference.

Intuitive communication has added a whole new dimension to these situations—from knowing what animals are thinking and feeling to a different way of looking at things, and the best way to resolve the issue. The answers are there, waiting to be unlocked.

20

Emotional Dependence

THE WONDERS OF MEDICAL INTUITION CAN GO FAR BEYOND the bounds of treating the physical side of animals. It can reach into the mental, emotional and spiritual beginnings of illnesses and injuries. Once one of these other aspects has been addressed, physical symptoms can disappear. I've seen it happen so many times, and it never fails to take my breath away.

One instance of this I experienced was when Avril emailed me in desperation about her cat, Bella. She had been scratching and tirelessly pulling her fur out. Avril had sought the help of several medical experts over this crisis, but they'd treated Bella mostly for allergy-related problems. This was to no avail, and the poor little thing's condition persisted over several months. Bella, a short-haired, sleek, black domestic cat, was an extremely intuitive and intelligent feline, mature beyond her young years. She conveyed to me that she always put Avril's needs ahead of her own, but now she'd reached breaking point.

Bella told me that there were disruptions going on at the house. She showed me a picture of a workman carrying tools and large planks of wood. Expanding my awareness I could hear hammering and drills in the background. It sounded like those on a construction site. Bella explained there were consistently loud strange noises, different smells and strangers wandering around. She also showed me many different people coming and going, who weren't workmen.

Bella didn't understand why all this commotion was necessary. She wanted to know what these people were doing in her house, and how long this would last. I felt her anxiety. I just knew how stressful all this felt to her, and that she no longer had harmony in her home. It was causing her body to rebel. Bella indicated she just needed quiet time alone with Avril, and that she wanted the bedroom door to be left open so she had a sanctuary when needing to retreat.

I relayed this to Avril, who confirmed that she was renovating and that she'd also recently started teaching classes at home, which explained the many people coming and going. Avril was relieved the issue wasn't of a physical nature and began making changes immediately. After a couple of weeks she phoned to say that once the renovations ceased, classes were confined to certain days and more time was spent with Bella, she couldn't believe the change in her cat. The skin irritation had completely cleared up. This physical condition clearly had come from an emotional cause.

There are many ways an animal can be suffering medically from emotional causes. For instance, it's very easy to project your own personality characteristics, feelings, thoughts and moods onto your animals, without realising it. This can greatly change an animal's behaviour. Projecting human-type attributes onto animals runs the risk of our no longer seeing those animals for who they truly are—we can end up treating them as mini-humans. This can become confusing for animals.

As traditional cultures are changing throughout the world, there are an increasing numbers of people turning to animals for 'family' support, often treating them as family members, friends or even, in some instances, life companions. The reality is that people (without intending to do so) utilise their companion animals to satisfy needs not met from human sources. Some may say that this is sad, but I'm not one of them, as long as the person doesn't become completely disenchanted with the human race.

Statistics show that, particularly in western cultures, the number of childless couples is increasing. For them, animals often act as child substitutes, and the lives of these couples are enriched by the qualities of love, nurturing and responsibility that occurs in these relationships. Animals have such giving natures, they're often lavished with love and indulgence. This is wonderful, as long as it isn't excessive.

Many animals are happy to share our lives, but not necessarily *become* our lives, if you know what I mean. They'd be far happier being themselves. It doesn't matter how kind your intentions, be careful that you don't only see *your* own perspective. As long as you are aware of the animal's needs also, this shouldn't be a problem. It comes back to mutual respect, and an understanding of the importance of moderation in all you do.

As an example, animals love attention, just as we do. But too much can create attention-seeking behaviour, as that's what they think you want. Separation anxiety can result. If you allow yourself to become such a big part of your animal's world, when you are not there, they find it difficult to cope. This is especially true for dogs, as they're pack animals and they come to see you as part of their pack. These animals are not used to doing things like playing by themselves or being on their own. A few hours seems like days to them and, for some, they feel like they're being punished, and they're not quite sure for what. It's all very puzzling for them and, at worst, they can work themselves up into such a state of anxiety that they injure themselves, for instance, by trying to get out of their backyard.

In a sense, we have taken away their independence and made them needy. That's why getting a grip on some of the basic laws of the jungle, if I can call them that, is so crucial for anyone who loves their cat or their dog. I don't have children, and at times do tend to be overprotective of my animals. I often ask myself if I impose my wants to cuddle and be needed onto them. It's an interesting and challenging question for anyone with an animal in their care.

Savannah, my small Japanese Spitz dog, broke her back leg when she was only six months old. It happened when she and I were out walking in the forest early one morning, along with my larger Japanese Spitz, Akeira. Both were on leashes when suddenly Akeira saw something run into the bushes. As she gave chase, Savannah followed, but being smaller she found it hard to keep up. I was struggling to contain both of them. Akeira came to a dead stop, and I did too, so as not to run into her. Unfortunately Savannah wasn't as quick to react and came to the end of her lead with a jerk. She yelped and huddled in a ball on the ground. As I ran over to her I knew something was seriously wrong.

The initial diagnosis at the vet's was a bad muscle strain in her back leg, but having these intuitive abilities gave me the strong sense of a break in her leg. I insisted she have an X-ray. Sure enough, there was a break in her left back leg. She underwent surgery and had to be confined to a holding cage for six weeks. I felt this was hard for dear little Savannah as she was a very energetic young dog who constantly wanted to play. Every day guilt would plague me, as I ran through in my mind whether or not I could have prevented her pain and anguish. I felt I was responsible for her coming to the end of her lead so abruptly. Every moment I could, I was squeezing and cuddling her tightly to reassure her everything would be all right.

In truth, she was absolutely fine and adapting to her confinement far better than I was. A few weeks after the accident Savannah communicated to me: *Mum, please, you are smothering me. I'm fine.* That I had been obsessing about her partially to ease my own guilt was a harsh realisation for me. I was showing her how sorry I was by holding her too close, as if asking her forgiveness. Savannah had no blame. She just wanted to get on with being a happy puppy. It was my inner sorrow that I was expressing, not hers.

The lesson here is that all of us, me included, have to watch that we don't over-obsess about our beloved animals. Memo to Trisha: lighten up!

I've learnt through experience with Mattie, my female Birman, that the big goodbye hug when I leave the house is for *my* benefit rather than hers. Mattie is very sophisticated and mature, and the face squeeze I had tried to give her every morning just wasn't her thing. It was as if she was saying, *Puh-lease, you're ruffling my coat.*

Mattie is my best friend and has been my main teacher of animal communication for years. In turn, I respect how she likes to be treated. She prefers a loving stroke and my telling her, 'See you tonight Mattie,' rather than having her face squeezed between my hands. We have a very close relationship and yes, she knows I love cuddles and, sweet girl that she is, will, on occasion, indulge me with her closeness, if only for a short time.

As I can communicate in their language and know my pets' specific likes and dislikes, there's no excuse for me to misunderstand their preferences. For me, like all us, it's about compromise between our needs and our animals' needs.

21

Animals Have Feelings

ANIMALS ARE SO LIKE US IN A MILLION WAYS. IT'S SUCH A PITY that often we don't get that. People assume certain animals have feelings and others don't. They think that fish just swim around their bowl or aquarium with little or no interaction with the other fish, when that's simply not the case.

Sophie contacted me about her Nemo, a male fish who looked exactly like Nemo from the movie. Sophie was concerned because her other similar fish, a female, was much larger and quite menacing. Sophie called her Queen Sheba, as she swam around the aquarium as though she owned it, while Nemo hovered by the water filter, as if trying to hide when Sheba swam by. If he ventured out she'd chase him back to the water filter.

When communicating with Queen Sheba I sensed a really dominant nature. She definitely liked being queen of the tank. I asked her why she felt she needed to prove her dominance. Even though Sheba assured me she wouldn't harm Nemo, she explained he was an adolescent and needed to be taught the rules of hierarchy. Wow! It seems the good old pecking order so favoured by humans is alive and well below the sea.

Speaking to Nemo, you could sense a much younger and gentler manner. He explained that Sheba's threatening nature always caused him to retreat. He didn't feel he could stand up to her as he was not aggressive by nature, and didn't want to pretend to be forceful. He told me he'd really like some other fish in the tank for back-up, preferably males, as he thought females may side with the queen. He'd previously been with Sheba in the aquarium at the shop and he knew that most of the fish in that tank were afraid of her. She wasn't, however, as dominant then as she was now.

After I'd explained the situation to Sophie she went out and bought another male fish. She decided to call him Salty and hoped a friendship would develop between him and Nemo. As soon as Salty entered the tank he was extremely inquisitive of the other fish, and being quite forthright he bowled straight up to the Queen and Nemo to investigate. Within days, Nemo and Salty were swimming around the tank together, with Nemo feeling more fearless with Salty at his side. Even Queen Sheba seemed to like the new arrangement. Perhaps she felt she had more subjects to rule! Things soon settled down and the three fish were able to go about their lives harmoniously.

Life being what it is, there are heaps of unavoidable events which can also cause emotional upsets for both animals and people. Pregnancy and the arrival of the new baby into a home certainly create a huge change in a household, and can cause stress and upset to your animal's life. Such was the case with Charmayne and her five-year-old King Charles Spaniel, Rusty.

Charmayne was eight months' pregnant and had noticed a considerable change in Rusty. He was being very disobedient in everything he was asked to do, sitting over to one side of the room as if to sulk. Charmayne was concerned as this was totally out of character for him. He was normally a loveable, happy dog, always willing to please and seldom naughty.

Rusty had had such a close relationship with Charmayne and they were rarely apart. One of their favourite activities had been their daily trip to the park where he'd have a swim in the lake. Then, at the end of an energetic day, Rusty would sleep at the bottom of the bed in between Charmayne and her husband Ryan. It was a blissful life for a pooch.

My talks with Rusty revealed that he felt Charmayne didn't love him anymore, because they rarely went out to the park these days, or on any outings for that matter. Rusty also said that he was now made to sleep *beside* the bed—not on it—which had never happened before. Rusty was sad because Charmayne seemed to be forever yelling at him. When I questioned his disobedience, he spoke of being confused at what was expected of him now. He was desperate to gain her attention, as it seemed to be fading.

Charmayne had tears streaming down her face as I passed on Rusty's responses to my questions. Rusty was her companion for most of the time as her husband was in the corporate world and spent much of his day at the office. She'd had no idea he was feeling so bereft. As she wiped her eyes, Charmayne explained that the pregnancy had made her very tired and irritable, and all she could do most days was just flop on the couch. She was very uncomfortable at this stage in her pregnancy so for Rusty to sit on her lap or sleep with her was not possible. Charmayne also admitted that at times it was all too much, and she became irritated at the slightest things.

My recommendation was for her to clearly visualise what she wanted from Rusty. This would help stop the confusion of mixed signals he was receiving. To try to avoid taking out her frustrations on him and to be patient, as the changes in her life were also affecting him. My final suggestion was to set aside time immediately for both of them to go to the park, or just to play together in the backyard.

Charmayne phoned me the next day to say she'd started all of my suggestions and, to her and her husband's amazement, Rusty had changed overnight. She thought it would be a slow process, but now realised that acknowledging his thoughts and feelings, and acting on them, had made such a big difference. He felt loved once more.

For Wilson, a rather large Great Dane, it wasn't a pregnancy that caused him to start acting weirdly. It was not until some time after the baby was born that he became particularly restless. Wilson took to running down to the back fence and hiding behind a tree. This became a daily practice and it concerned Greg and his wife Angela. They couldn't understand what was causing him to act this way.

Wilson had been a part of the family for six years, even before they were married. He was like their son, and was pampered as such; their gentle giant never seemed to grow up. Greg and Angela even took him on beach holidays with them where they all played games together and had a ball. Sharing the bed was a squeeze, but they managed!

Both Greg and Angela had made a big effort throughout her pregnancy, birth and beyond to keep things mostly the same for Wilson. They didn't want him to feel left out or no longer a part of the family as he always had been. It wasn't until Jasmine, their daughter, was around eighteen months old that things altered. Angela and Greg were now genuinely concerned, and they brought me in as they had many questions for Wilson.

The situation became very clear to me after the first couple of questions I asked him. He told me how much he loved Greg and Angela, and was wondering why they didn't trust him. Wilson showed me a little girl who he adored, but was never allowed to demonstrate his love to, or even to get close to her. He said, *Every time I try, I'm either pushed away or told to go sit at a distance.* He felt he was being punished and he just knew they didn't trust him. He couldn't believe that his mum and dad would think he would harm his sister. They didn't seem to know how much he loved her and wanted to play with her. He explained he could feel the anxiety within Angela every time he was near Jasmine. Wilson said, *I must be very bad for them to feel this way. Whenever Jasmine is brought outside, I run to the back of the house and behind the tree to show I will be good. I'm very hurt and embarrassed that they feel this way. I would never hurt her.*

My heart really went out to Wilson. Obviously there was a great misunderstanding going on here, and everyone was suffering. Greg and Angela just couldn't believe what I told them. They didn't think he was bad at all. Angela in particular felt guilty, as she tended to get tense when she placed Jasmine on the ground outside with Wilson, not because she thought he'd harm her, but because he is such a big dog: his tail wagging had even knocked her over a couple of times. They asked me what they could do to help this situation.

Firstly, I had to go back and explain to Wilson it was just his large stature and playfulness that was a little too much for someone as small as Jasmine, and that Greg and Angela didn't think he was bad at all—in fact they loved him very much. I needed to explain that he could eventually play more with Jasmine as she got bigger, but at the moment there had to be restrictions. I also advised Jasmine's parents to involve Wilson in games with her.

Wilson was watching her grow from a baby into a little girl and he loved her dearly. Obviously she had to be out of harm's way but, with supervision, Wilson could have limited contact which would give him a sense of involvement. It's amazing how much we learn when we look at situations from another's perspective.

22

New Environments

RELOCATING TO A DIFFERENT SUBURB, CITY OR COUNTRY CAN be extremely stressful for your animal. There's so much to organise, not to mention the packing and inconvenience. Your mind will be buzzing as you try to make sure you haven't forgotten to take care of finishing up everything at the old premises while getting things started at the new address. Although usually exciting, it can become quite a headache.

When the boxes are being packed and the house is in constant disarray over several weeks, you can just imagine how this might appear to your animal. They feel and see the disruption, but don't have a clue what it's all about. It can cause a lot of angst when their bed is in a totally different place or can't be found as it's been packed. Their meals and the times they're fed may have changed too, due to the upheaval. Throw into the mix the attention from their people reduced to a minimum because of the increase in your workload, and it's like having massive changes occur in your life without knowing why or how long they will last!

Cats seem to feel the stress of losing their home much more than other animals, such as dogs and birds. Dogs go for walks and travel in the car fairly frequently, so their environment does have variation. Many birds kept in aviaries or cages tend to have their home fully relocated with them, thereby minimising trauma. But cats don't normally get to visit unfamiliar environments often.

Relocation for an indoor cat is a complete change of what it knows and, even if your cat is an indoor/outdoor cat, the backyard and the neighbourhood are still part of its territory, so in many respects it has a lot to lose when its family moves. Think about it. It can take time for a cat to build up its territory, and it may have had to defend it from other cats, which may have led brutal fighting when doing so. Friendships may have been formed with other animals in the neighbourhood and cats that roam could also have other houses, structures and areas they like to visit. So cats will usually express their disapproval, before during and after any move.

There are definitely people who are aware of the distress moving house has on their animals, and those who know my work will often book a consultation with me before they relocate, as they want to make the change for their beloved animals with minimal stress. Carmen contacted me regarding Julius, her male Siamese cat, who was a confident, mature fellow. He hated having his routine disrupted. Carmen was about to begin the big pack up and had ordered removal boxes to arrive in the next day or so, and she knew Julius would then get wind that something big was going on. She wanted me to explain to Julius what was about to happen and how the relocation would affect him.

Their current house was in a quiet area with natural bushland behind their property, allowing Julius the freedom of a large territory where he could roam and hunt for small mice. He was quite the hunter, enjoying this as part of his daytime activity. It wasn't very far to their new place, but it was in a more suburban setting on a busier road. Carmen wanted to find out how he would feel about this. She wanted him to understand that it would be better if he confined himself to the backyard in the new place and not venture out the front for she feared he would be run over. Carmen also asked if there was anything she could do that would make it easier for him.

In no uncertain terms, Julius let me know that he wanted to roam wherever he pleased—he was more than capable of taking care of himself. Surprisingly, he asked me why humans felt the need for change, and why they're never satisfied. He couldn't understand why it was necessary to move at all. In his case, he reckoned life was perfectly fine where they were.

I did my best to point out that certain events come up in humans' lives that can make it necessary to shift to a different suburb, and that this upheaval, though it might be tough to begin with, can be beneficial to all concerned. I didn't sense Julius was fully convinced, but there was no doubt he wanted to go where his family was.

23

When Animals Mirror Humans

LIKE CHILDREN, ANIMALS TEND TO COPY OUR CHARACTERISTICS. They come into our lives at a very young age and they may identify with us instead of their own species. Relying mostly on non-verbal communication, animals are inclined to observe and read our body language far better than we do, so they will sometimes imitate even the most subtle of human actions and reactions. They can also mirror the mental and emotional states of their human companions, both positive and negative.

The behaviour of an animal can be a direct reflection of the actions and attitudes of those in their human environment. Over the years I have seen how the personality of the person who raises an animal has a direct bearing on who that animal is. The same as it is with people. Anxious people tend to have anxious animals. Playful, happy people tend to have the same sort of animals. It's not always an exact science, but certainly has been prominently borne out in all the work I've done.

We learn that it is always safe to love an animal, as they just love us for who we truly are. For some people, this may be the only time they have experienced unconditional love. If you totally depend on your animal for all the love in your life, or constantly smother them, the animal will try to fill your needs and may even abandon their own needs in favour of yours, becoming totally dependent on you. This is not healthy for the animal or you.

There have been times in my life, especially as a child, when life seemed devoid of the love I was craving. My parents were having their own problems and there didn't seem to be a lot of attention thrown my way. I relied on my companion animals, including our dog Slasher, a fiercely loyal and protective friend. His unconditional love set the scene for our strong relationship and taught me to be less judgemental of others. I tended to favour his nature over most of the humans I interacted with. He was kind and gentle and didn't have an aggressive bone in his body. We were inseparable. Whenever I wasn't in school I'd sit and talk to him for hours, discussing my thoughts and dilemmas. He sat and listened intently and patiently. Willingly, he gave me the attention I so craved.

While I was at school, Slasher would go off wandering for hours at a time and, no matter how we secured the backyard, he kept escaping—although he was always back in time to greet me upon my return. I now realise he had needs of his own, and he pursued these when we were apart. He liked to go and visit the men at the ice works a couple of streets away. They'd feed him treats, play ball and rough and tumble with him, as guys do. This was quite different from our relationship. It taught me that not all our needs are the same. We require a variety of things and different relationships to fulfill our lives.

Animals can get caught up in people's imbalances because of their great desire to please and help, and sickness or behavioural issues can result when the animal attempts to take away misery from us. It can prove too big a burden for them. At times they'll even mirror the particular issue their person is experiencing. It's their attempt to help us understand what's going on with our emotional and physical bodies.

Helena, was concerned about the health of her cat, Leah, an extremely beautiful five-year-old part-Persian with insulin-dependent diabetes. She wanted me to ask Leah how the condition was affecting her, and also to intuitively scan her body for extra medical information. Leah explained to me how at times she experienced light-headedness and nausea. Helena later confirmed Leah would urgently need to eat at certain times of the day, which these symptoms demanded.

When scanning Leah's body I sensed abdominal pain in the kidneys and liver and that the level of her urea (a by-product of the liver) was high. Helena verified that Leah had permanent damage to her liver with her last tests showing the urea at high levels.

It was, however, the latter part of my conversation with Leah that was a bit more disturbing. She wanted me to ask Helena to relax more, as she was constantly stressed and worried about the rest of the family. Leah said that the other members weren't very supportive of Helena, even though she was unwell. Leah wanted to share the illness with Helena, to be that vital support she needed. She didn't want Helena going through it on her own, and hoped Helena would review her own illness. I was touched by how unselfish and compromising Leah was but puzzled that she thought Helena was unwell.

When I questioned Helena about her health she told me that she had diabetes too, and she was indeed neglecting herself. She was looking after her elderly mother, which I suppose kind of gave her permission to ignore her own wellbeing.

Leah had certainly done what she had set out to do. It definitely made Helena stop and think about herself more— and that if she was healthier, then Leah would be too. It never ceases to amaze me the sacrifices animals are prepared to make for us.

As I mentioned earlier, animals may mirror events through their behaviour. This was the case with Gypsy, a brightly coloured, exotic parrot. She was housed in a large metal cage inside the home of Talia and her son, Brian. Talia had been a single parent for the past ten years, ever since her husband had left for another woman and denied all responsibility for Brian, who was eight years old at the time.

Life hadn't been easy for Talia, with the emotional and financial responsibility of her son, and living her life without a partner. And it hadn't been easy for Brian either, not only growing up without a father throughout some of the most impressionable years of his life but also always feeling, deep down, he'd done something wrong to lose the love of his father. Brian had now become a rebellious teenager, which was a quite a challenge for Talia.

Already under a lot of strain, Talia couldn't cope when Gypsy took to screeching at the top of her lungs for no apparent reason. Thinking Gypsy was in pain she took her to the vet, but everything was fine. Talia told me that a few months before Gypsy began screeching whenever Brian or his male friends entered the room when Talia was there too. The the high pitched cry was almost deafening.

When I turned up and chatted with Gypsy, this unbelievable bird made it clear that whenever Brian or his friends were in the room with Talia, he was mimicking the tones she heard. Gypsy explained the pitch and the anxiety level were high. It happened so much that she was not only mimicking, but also protesting at the tension and noise. Gypsy showed me images of Talia and Brian in full verbal abuse, engaged in arguments that were very intense and which often involved his friends. Poor Gypsy felt she had no alternative but to show them what they were doing to each other, and what she too was enduring.

I was careful when I gave Talia the low-down on Gypsy's behaving so strangely, because this was a sensitive issue. It's a problem that is difficult to avoid in such strained circumstances, but one that needed to be resolved.

Talia was speechless, not having previously realised that these arguments with Brian were so severe and, more to the point, that they occurred more often than not. She felt guilty, as she was the adult and she wasn't handling the situation well. She couldn't believe she had put Gypsy through this trauma.

I wanted to point out to Talia that raising a child on her own was an amazing feat in itself. Rather than taking the blame she should, I suggested, forgive herself and, perhaps, see a counsellor for herself and Brian to resolve the many issues they faced. It took one beautiful girl, Gypsy, to bring about a full recovery. Arguing rarely solves anything . . . just ask Gypsy.

These forms of mirroring are extremely important and shouldn't be taken lightly. They are an animal's way of showing us how we're behaving or, in a health situation, what we need. They're silent observers and will often see more about us than we do. More significantly, they are truthful observers.

If we don't want to admit something to ourselves, we tend to ignore it. Animals see it and display it as it really is. If they're mirroring you, then there is something really vital they need you to acknowledge. To ignore the messages they're giving us is to miss out on real enlightenment. And don't forget that *their* suffering is likely to continue indefinitely if we turn away from their cries from the heart.

PART IV

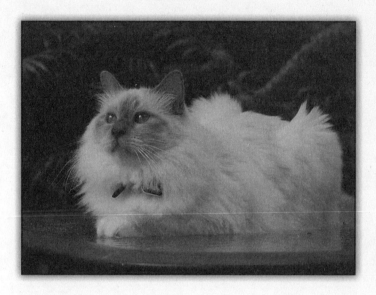

Animals Are Not Human

24

Living in a Human World

IF YOU WANT THE BEST FOR YOUR ANIMALS, THEN YOU NOT only need to love them but also to pay close attention to ensure they get everything they require to be truly happy and healthy. This includes taking their diet seriously. The days of giving them leftovers off your plates and leaving it at that are over—it's not good enough. Without proper care and attention to their nutritional needs animals suffer.

Take the story of Melinda, who contacted me regarding Sunny, her Poodle. She was worried about his diet because he wouldn't eat his greens. Sunny was a no-nonsense dog. If he didn't like something he displayed this very clearly. (I know plenty of humans who'd take Sunny's side on the issue of eating vegetables!) Melinda wondered if I could ask him why he didn't like them. So I communicated with this outspoken Poodle, only to find out that it wasn't as simple as him not liking vegetables.

Sunny saw himself as equal in standing to his family and didn't see why *he* should have to eat anything Melinda and her husband didn't eat. He'd preferred to eat what *they* were eating and, anyway, they often shared food with him from their own plates. Where did this come from—his personality, or bad habits?

When I discussed the situtation with Melinda, she looked a little red-faced. She told me she and her husband quite often grabbed a take-away meal on their way home from work, which didn't include much vegetable and, yes, they shared it with Sunny because he wouldn't eat his meals. Melinda had her answer.

There has been a great deal of scientific study to show how a regime as close to nature as possible keeps animals fitter and healthier, allowing them to live longer and need fewer visits to the vet. Animals are closely linked to nature, so it stands to reason they'll respond well to an eating regime that's natural. If you compare your pet with similar creatures in the wild, you'll find that undomesticated critters have a raw diet and regular exercise. You should consider your animal's diet and activities. They're more crucial than you think.

And here's the bonus: helping them to be healthy will help your wellbeing as it connects you to what's natural. I can't stress strongly enough just how significant this is, and how great the rewards can be for both you and your animal.

I'm sad to say that the amount of different cancers I see in young animals is nothing short of astonishing. Some are in animals as young as three years old. Various cancers, along with certain other diseases, have been linked to poor or inadequate diets in people; we know this is true. Through my work I'm now seeing many of the same diseases in humans turning up in animals at an increasingly alarming rate. Perhaps the animals are trying to show us what we need to look at in our own lifestyles in order to prevent these diseases.

The pressure of animals wanting us to give them unhealthy food can be eliminated if they're only given *healthy* foods. When people introduce them to unhealthy scraps from the table, as well as sugary treats, they begin craving these foods. Humans do exactly the same. If we had never been introduced to extremely salty, sugary or fatty and processed foods, we wouldn't miss them. That is why you start your animals on a healthy raw diet—if it's what they're used to, then it's what they'll eat.

Dogs are predominantly meat eaters and have their particular teeth and bowel types to cope with this diet. Their teeth are for ripping and tearing meat, and their bowels are perfectly designed to digest meat. Wild dogs don't cook their meat after killing an animal or finding a dead carcass. They eat raw meat. That's what keeps them healthy. Cooked meat may start to appeal to them if they get a taste for it, but it's not natural. There's also a chemical reaction in food once it's been cooked and food that is charred or burnt may be potentially carcinogenic. Dogs will also consume grasses, herbs and berries in the wild, and there is also a degree of vegetable matter eaten when they consume the stomach contents of their prey.

Unhealthy foods can make an animal very fussy about its diet. How do you solve this? The reality is that you have to be cruel to be kind, or your animal might end up in all sorts of trouble. If you're concerned about your dog's or cat's vitamin and mineral intake, there are plenty of many natural food supplements available. Raw meaty bones (never cooked as that makes them too brittle) should be the bulk of their diet, or full carcasses wherever possible. The ripping and tearing of meat for dogs and cats are essential for the health of their teeth and gums. Chicken necks or wings will provide them with the bone content, and help to clean their teeth naturally. Larger bones are perfect for larger animals.

Remember, though, never to leave animals unattended with bones, as they can occasionally get stuck on their teeth or in their throats. I have on rare occasions had to retrieve a piece of chicken neck from the molar or the throat of Mattie and Shea, emergencies which frightened the heck out of both me and them!

Most commonly found canned foods, especially those sold at the supermarkets, have preservatives and additives. These can be extremely unhealthy to give animals and many contain foods that wouldn't normally be in their natural diets. They can also be highly addictive, so animals begin to crave them in their diet. Like the meals offered in most fast-food chains, masses of sugar and salt are added to get them hooked.

Most people wouldn't like to be the cause of ill health in their beloved animal companions. For both our animals and ourselves, going natural and chemical free would minimise disease. Just as chemicals are contributing to the ill health in people, so it contributes to illnesses in our animal companions. Think about what's best for them and their health. Be strict with yourself as well for the same reasons. Like us, an animal with the proper diet and plenty of exercise will be healthy and happy for a long time to come.

25

A Cat's Life

CATS, LIKE DOGS, ARE CARNIVORES, WHICH MEANS THEY ALSO require mostly meat in their diet. In the wild, they'd eat whole carcasses of prey. At home try replicating this as much as possible. No, that doesn't mean you need to go out with a bow and arrow and kill something—that's why we have supermarkets and butchers.

In order to be healthy and happy, cats require a substance in meats, particularly red meats, called taurine. If your cats love the outdoors you will know how quickly they take any opportunity to catch lizards, mice or rats, allowing them to supply themselves with fresh meat, not to mention the thrill of the chase. I can't stress enough the importance of fresh meat—preferably organic or from the butcher—for cats. If the meat is ripe, though, they'll more than likely reject this offering, which is funny given that dogs will dig something up after days or weeks of festering and still consider it a delicacy!

You should also add livers, kidneys or other offal periodically to a cat's diet, along with a very small amount of vegetables every couple of days, which they would obtain naturally in the wild from the stomach contents of their prey. And don't forget to leave out a fresh supply of water every day for all your animals—filtered if possible. Filtered may sound like an extravagance, but many cats have told me they'd rather not drink water that smells of chlorine or other chemicals. Fussy as they are, clean, fresh water is best for them.

Keep in mind too that if your animal has a medical condition, then their diet may need adjusting, so discuss this with your vet. In most cases there are usually natural alternatives to packaged food to cover any concerns you may have.

Cats also need stimulation and exercise. Of course it would be wonderful if they were free to roam with relative safety wherever they wanted to go. But suburban or apartment living makes it difficult for our feline friends to wander the neighbourhood. This is why many cats are confined to a house or yard. There are many dangers out there that aren't built into a cat's instinct, such as cars and swimming pools, and even people who dislike animals and set out to cause them harm. In the wild, they'd have open spaces and trees to climb if they needed an urgent escape. It's different in backyards because, if a cat is confronted by a menacing dog, there mightn't be any tree to scale and the fence could be too high.

Cat-runs, although not offering complete freedom, enable them to come and go from the house, giving them choice and a sense of freedom. Cats love to view things from great heights, so these runs should be built up high using a fence for support or attached to part of the house. This love is due to their feline nobility—without doubt cats like looking down on us.

Cat mesh encompassing the whole yard is another way of containing them, and keeping unwanted animals out. It also provides important safety for birds or other wildlife from cats. And if you're in an apartment, then a window ledge with a protective flyscreen is a must. But be careful about allowing cats on balconies as there have been many bones broken, as well as fatalities, when cats fall from an unnatural height. They may have been distracted by a fast-flying bird, or drifted off during one of their cat naps, and disaster followed.

Fresh air and sunlight are vital for the wellbeing of cats, just as it is for us. You can take them to a park or simply let them out in your backyard on a harness, for them to roam and explore. Of course this will require your supervision. The first time Peter and I took Mattie and Shea to the park on a harness, the looks from other people were priceless. They probably thought at first that they were dogs—until they got close enough to see they were actually cats. I'm sure they thought we were quite mad.

Within your home you can provide a play area with nooks and crannies for your cat, including a scratchy pole. If you want your cat to leave your furniture alone, you *must* give them a scratchy pole as they need to scratch to remove the outer casing of their nails. Cats outside scratch up against trees daily for this reason; it is fundamental for them.

Cat tunnels for them to hide in are another form of play and stimulation and this is a joy for humans to watch. There's nothing they love more than leaping out at you with the element of surprise and grabbing an ankle in the fun of things. I confess Shea brings me down to my knees on occasions when he shoots out of his tunnel like a cannonball. He is always so proud of himself, of course, as I am left trying to get to my feet.

Hanging cat toys around or providing small balls will amuse them but, most importantly, having you play with them is a must. You'll have a ball, and create a playmate for each other. I feel *I* have more fun than Mattie and Shea in our playtimes, which rather suggests I'm just a big kid at heart! Swinging a furry mouse from side to side and then watching the amazing heights my cats reach with their acrobatics is a delight for me. There's a particular game I play with them, where my hand acts like a claw, and as I play it their body language dramatically changes. Their pupils dilate, they make this huffing sound with their nostrils and they adopt a 'ready to pounce' stance. It then comes down to speed and accuracy, between them and me. Of course they always win, and I'm left licking my wounds—pride that is, not blood.

If you have several cats and they get on well together, like Mattie and Shea do, then this will provide them with their own enjoyment. Just like dogs, any bored or unstimulated cat will probably develop unwanted behaviours, like ruining furniture or urinating on various things in your home. This is how cats express themselves. Try not to get too angry at them. Your cat is trying to tell you something needs resolving.

They are after all, simply being cats.

26

Obesity Problems

IN A PERFECT WORLD WE'D ALL BE PHYSICALLY, EMOTIONALLY AND spiritually balanced. Becoming self-sufficient is one way of attaining balance. The flipside is that relying totally on others for our love or confidence can make life very unstable. Deep down we know that not everyone in our lives is reliable, or has honorable intentions. In short: the best kind of love needs to come from within ourselves.

Animals are great teachers in helping us to love ourselves, but if we are full of self-loathing, sometimes the fallout can affect our beloved animals too. There's no doubt that we cannot survive without love. Imagine never having experienced love from your parents, siblings or a partner in life. For some, this experience is real. That is why so many people will look elsewhere for the love they so crave. It can be in the form of addictions, such as food used as comfort for unsatisfied emotions. It's a way of filling the void. But as they get solace from this, the habits often transfer to their animals.

As it is in humans, obesity in animals is on the increase, and I'm seeing it all the time in my practice. If you look at the journey through past generations there are some obvious changes in the health of animals, as well as humans. As animals become more a part of our lifestyle, there is the danger of loving your animals too much. You may like to indulge and pamper them, for their amazing understanding and support, by giving them sugary treats from your table and generally overfeeding them (albeit mostly out of affection). Well, perhaps animals are, once again, trying to show us what we're doing to ourselves.

You'd have to be blind not to see the damage caused by obesity and the prevailing medical conditions that follow. It can lead to painful life-threatening illnesses and a shorter lifespan for our dear animals, as it does for us. These risks can include pancreatitis and kidney and liver disease, as well as heart and circulatory disorders, arthritis from the strain on various joints, an increase in surgical and anaesthetic risks, and skin disorders. Yikes! It's alarming, isn't it?

When animals are ill we go to great lengths to heal them, but helping them find their way out of obesity will also assist us to adopt a better diet and exercise regime for ourselves. We have all become so distracted with our busy lives that we're not making space for ourselves and our development. And if we have no regard for ourselves, what time do we make available for the much-loved animal companions who share our lives? When our animals are constantly pleading for food, it isn't necessarily food they want—but attention.

As mentioned earlier, I admit I'm far stricter with the diet of my beloved animals than I am with my own. Even though I've always been relatively slim, the older I get, the more I have to watch what I eat. As their carer, I'm very aware of my responsibility towards them, and make sure they have a proper diet available. They can't get their own food so they rely on me to make the correct choices. It's when they look at you with those big soulful eyes, or place a loving lick on your hand, that your willpower is forced to its limit. It would be easy to give in to those you love so dearly. Unfortunately one treat turns into many, as I have found out personally.

We often don't notice that our animals have put on weight, as it's usually so gradual, just like us. All of a sudden they are very overweight—but take heart, there are many practical things we can do to prevent or reduce the problem. By the time people come seeking my help with their overweight dogs and cats, they're looking for solutions. They usually know they're guilty of overindulgence, but find it hard to stop the habit, as the animal looks so sad if refused food. I'm sure you would too if someone took your favourite indulgence away. But when I look into my animal's eyes, I want to feel sure I'm not shortening their life in any way.

27

Fat Cats and Dogs

MOST OF THE CONSULTATIONS I'M CALLED IN ON REGARDING obesity issues are usually by owners who ask me to explain to their animal friend why they need to have their food restricted. This was the case for Marcus, a cute Golden Retriever. Georgina, who cared for Marcus, wanted me to tell him why they needed to stop feeding him treats or food from their plates. Georgina wasn't the only one who was guilty of overfeeding, as she lived with her mother, Freda, who couldn't resist Marcus either. Georgina wanted him to know he was much loved, but that she feared for his health.

As you can imagine the reply wasn't that different to what you'd expect from a human under similar circumstances. Marcus was an adorable puppy-like dog, even though he was eight years old. He was very affectionate and loved attention, always longing for a dog companion, as he had a lot of energy to expel and was prone to boredom. Georgina and Freda became his world.

Marcus had been obese for so long that having these additional tidbits was a habit, a habit he didn't particularly want to break. He was so used to getting what he wanted *when* he wanted it. But it wasn't so much the food, more the patting and attention he received with the treats. Marcus liked feeling important and being a part of the family, and eating and doing the things *they* did. When I asked Marcus if he was actually hungry at those times, after a little hesitation, he replied with, *No not really*.

I explained to him that this extra food would have to stop for health reasons, and that it would be done so gradually he'd hardly notice. He seemed disappointed but knew in time things would be fine. I then suggested to Georgina and Freda they take him out for more walks and games for exercise. Shamed-faced, they admitted they had been quite slack in that area. There would be no more extra treats or feeding from their plates. He would be fed two smaller meals a day, with one small treat at the end of exercise. I also suggested he be praised and given lots of attention around exercise and also at non-feeding times.

Georgina sounded a little skeptical, although she understood what had to be done. She contacted me several weeks later to say she was delighted with his weight loss, and that she now had a more energetic dog. He had been sad at first with the restrictions, but was now happier and healthier. Georgina felt he didn't notice the lack of extra food any more, and very much looked forward to walk times with her and Freda. She was very proud of herself. She'd seen it through, and now knew she was in charge of his health, and hers. Through all that walking, she couldn't believe how much energy she had also, not to mention Freda.

When animals have been obese for a long time, the habit definitely becomes ingrained, and can be more difficult to break. If the animal has only been overweight for a relatively short time, things can be easier. A gorgeous long-haired tortoiseshell feline named Mirella is a perfect example.

Shelly contacted me regarding two-year-old Mirella's weight gain, which she'd only noticed recently. While I was questioning Shelly about Mirella's feeding habits, I discovered that she had started a new job six months earlier, and now she and her husband, Martin, led such busy lives that their eating habits were less than perfect. Shelly had begun feeding Mirella the same food they were eating, as it was quicker and easier, and Mirella didn't seem to mind.

Mirella was a placid cat, tending to always fit in with her persons. She loved to lie in the sun during the day and would choose a prime spot on the couch at night next to Shelly.

When I questioned Mirella about her diet I was quite surprised. She told me she craved raw red meat like she used to get, and that she didn't really like the taste of this new food. But that was what she was offered, so she complied. Mirella complained of stomach upset and feeling lethargic. She didn't like either of these sensations and asked if I could make them go away.

I promised that her diet would now go back to raw meat, which would taste better and help her to lose her weight. I asked her to trust me: I promised that before long she'd feel her energy return.

Shelly felt she had let Mirella down and was keen to get her back to a healthier diet. She also realised that being busy was no excuse for an unhealthy diet for herself and Martin either. Shelly came up with some time-saving ways of pre-

preparing healthy meals and freezing them. Mind you, I didn't want her to be too hard on herself, as things in life do change and this can make good choices more difficult. Just like us, animals can crave fatty or salty food but the difference is they don't know the dangers of these additives.

Shelly contacted me several months later and confessed it had taken her a couple of weeks to get organised into the new routine. But she was pleased to report that Mirella had lost most of her excess weight, and that she and her husband's diet was far better now as well.

Our love for our animals' wellbeing does have a very big impact on ours too. Shelly's story is yet another example.

28

Weight-loss Tips

HERE'S SOME SUGGESTIONS TO ASSIST ANIMALS WITH THEIR weight loss. For this to work you need to change their diet and exercise regimes. But please, before you start, it's a good idea to consult your vet in case of any medical problems.

Diet

- Do not feed your animal friends from your plate. This initiates bad habits.
- Try to ignore those big eyes looking back at you pleading for more food, and try to ignore those increasingly loud yowls from felines. This should eventually stop.
- Please try to restrain your urge to give treats as a sign of love. Instead, substitute a walk, a massage or other healthy activity.
- Feed wholesome, natural, raw food. If they are overweight, reduce the amounts you give them slowly over two to three weeks. In some cases a dietary food may be required for extremely overweight animals.

- Feed smaller portions throughout the day as this can help your animal feel full.
- Keep filtered water available for them at all times.
- If you have several animals, but only one is affected by obesity, then feed that animal away from the others. He or she doesn't want to feel like you're punishing them when they see the others eating differently. Also, it might create aggression if the obese animals feels they have to compete with the others in the house for food.
- Regularly weigh or examine your animal companion for weight loss, so you can see if your hard work is paying off. If you're doing all the correct things and your animal friend is not losing any weight, then consult your vet.
- Don't ever leave excess or extra food out so the animal can eat whenever it wants. The food needs to be restricted to meal times only.
- Most of all be patient, as with all weight loss it will take time, and they need your support to get to their goal weight.

Think about it: exercising your four-legged friend mostly involves you. Yes, they may play with other animals or entertain themselves briefly with toys but, as their constant companion and guardian, it's your responsibility to make sure they keep active with adequate exercise and play. I'm sure *you* could do with a bit more exercise as well. This can be great fun.

Exercise
- If your animal is extremely obese, then keep exercise to a moderate level done in shorter bursts. As fitness kicks in, you can increase the duration and the intensity.

- Provide plenty of water throughout exercise.
- Swimming should be utilised where possible, as this is kinder on the joints.
- Social interaction with other animals is a must, as it's a natural form of exercise.
- Make sure this exercise is daily (animals *and* you!).
- When exercising cats, use toys you can move quickly, or remote-controlled toys. They love attacking feathers, or fast-moving objects, as it stimulates and exercises them. Think like a cat and be very creative.

Our animal companions are definitely members of our family. We love them and want to keep them safe and healthy, so it's important we keep them fit, not fat. The next time your animal wants to play, stop what you're doing and invest in the relationship with your best friend. Friendships and relationships take time and commitment to make them as rewarding and enriching as possible.

29

Caring for Cats

ANIMALS MOULT, AND THIS IS A NATURAL PART OF PREPARING FOR a new season. They don't wear clothes but they need their coats to vary in thickness to accommodate climatic changes. The dear things can't remove their fur coat at the end of winter like we do but, rather, have to shed it over time. I know this is irritating, but animals don't have a choice, so cut them some slack if this is upsetting you.

True, certain dogs and cats don't shed their fur but you'll find these breeds aren't as tolerant to temperature change. You must keep this in mind because some of these animals should have their hair or fur shaved to give them comfort in hot conditions.

Now for a housekeeping tip—although, what I'm about to say is housekeeping with a spiritual upside! Sharing our lives with cats means that a good vacuum system is a must, because cat fur manages to get into every corner of the house.

I know it can be annoying, but you'll be fascinated to know that even something as simple as a cat shedding fur can have a symbolic meaning for us. It signifies shedding stuff we no longer need in our lives—the letting go of the so many things we cling to that no longer serve us. In my opinion, 'letting go' can set us free. It's big stuff.

Imagine if cats hung onto all the extra fur they no longer needed. They'd overheat in summer and become extremely unwell. Applying that to our own lives, there's a stage when we have to get rid of the old to make way for the new. It is the only way to progress.

As you've no doubt observed, felines can tend to come across as very select about who they spend time with. Yes, they're extremely loyal, but you can't force them to be affectionate. They're also extremely dignified in their approach and can be reserved but, curiously, although appearing aloof, they have told me that they do love us to share in their cat world.

There have been many occasions when I've been standing in the bathroom fixing my hair or cleaning my teeth and Shea will come and sit very closely beside my foot. I look down and will find him grooming his back leg and lying it across my foot, so I can be involved in his grooming. At times when I'm lying on the bed, 'Mattie the Queen', as I call her, will join me, and she too will lie close. There have been occasions in her grooming where she will be licking her paw, then *my* hand, and back to her paw again. I feel extremely privileged, not only to share in their world, but that they choose to care and nurture me to this degree. Even though their raspy tongues can cause a little discomfort! It's their way of expressing love.

One of the qualities a cat has that is not shared by any other animal is their ability to purr, and this mesmerising sound has amazing healing qualities, due to its wave frequency, or vibration. It's even been found to lower blood pressure and relieve breathing disorders in humans. Just hearing their purr makes you more relaxed and loved, as cats usually only purr when they are content.

It won't surprise you to know that I regard cats as one of the great joys in the world. I see them as a gift of the highest order. Whether it's cats in domesticity, or those in the wild, they have so much to teach us—beginning with their inherent credo that it's the simple things in life that create the greatest happiness. They have this amazing insight, and they can impart it, as long as we're open to the spiritual adventure.

When cats use their claws on one of the dining room chairs, they don't know it's your beloved furniture they're scratching, so don't be too cross with them. To them, your highly valued chairs are just pieces of wood, and they can't think of a single reason not to scratch away to their heart's content. As I've said before, cats need to regularly remove the outer casing of their nails. If they can't find wood, then coarse fabrics such as curtains and couches will suffice, irrespective of how much you may treasure them. However, if you provide them with a suitable scratchy pole, or scratching device, you can encourage them to use this.

Here's a tip you'll love me for when you see how well it works: when you see them scratching your belongings, take them to the scratchy pole and gently hold their front paws and run their claws down the rope or carpet on the pole. Cats will soon catch on that this is where they scratch. The pole should be sturdy and contain varied materials for the best results. Make sure it's a reasonable size too, as your cat needs to be able to fully stretch and reach up this pole, like they would a tree. And it needs to be accessible. There's no point it being in a spare room with the door shut. Cats love having something that is theirs, that they can lie on, scratch and play with, whenever the mood takes them, especially an indoor cat, where trees are not an option.

A gorgeous rag doll cat called Jessica began scratching the couch and the dining room setting of the home she shared with Janelle. The cat was normally very placid but didn't like change, and had a tendency of liking her own way. Janelle couldn't understand why, after many years of using her scratchy pole, Jessica had switched to leaving her mark on anything and everything.

Jessica communicated to me that her precious scratchy pole had been moved to another room and wasn't as accessible. She liked it in its usual spot as it was easy to get to in the main living area where the rest of her human family spent time. Jessica liked to be near them. Being shifted to another room made her feel forgotten and out of the way. Jessica also felt that perhaps she didn't hold the same importance any more. When Janelle moved the scratchy pole back to its original place, Jessica once again only used her rope pole for her claws.

Cats will often communicate with their urine. If they need to get a message across to you, they'll use urine in what we humans consider inappropriate places, like on your best couch or on the curtains. Faeces will be deposited to leave a message of grave importance. If a cat is displaying territorial behaviour or protecting itself, then it will do these things to set a clear boundary for unwanted visitors. While we hate this, it's natural for cats to do it.

Marcus and Judith wanted me to find out why their pure white Persian cat, Snow, had begun spraying the couch and the curtains with urine. He was a neutered indoor cat and this trouble had only started recently. The curtains he targeted were the ones hanging over the sliding glass door which led to the back patio. Judith had washed the couch and curtains several times in a special solution to remove the smell but, no matter how many times she washed everything, Snow would re-spray them.

This was extremely unusual for Snow as he was nine years old and had always been an unobtrusive character. He was usually content to curl up in his bed or on the couch for most of the day. He seemed to be acting completely out of character and Marcus and Judith were very concerned at this sudden shift, in case he wasn't well.

When I communicated with Snow, he was extremely gentle and quite willing to talk. We got on really well. This situation had been bothering him for some time and he was busting to explain what was happening. Snow felt Marcus and Judith had the wrong idea about his recent antics. He showed me a picture of a large ginger-and-white male cat who had been coming into the yard at night, toileting in the garden and then sleeping for several hours under the patio near the sliding glass doors. Snow showed me this cat looking right back at him through the glass. Snow felt threatened and needed to deter this cat from coming into his territory. He couldn't do this outside as he was an indoor cat. So he sprayed the curtains and the couch, as they were the closest to the back door, to let the other cat know he was invading someone else's territory.

Judith and Marcus had no idea this was the cause, or that a big male cat was coming by each evening and acting in such a menacing way. They promptly swung into action, spending the next few nights regularly turning the back light on and venturing out through the glass doors to scare away any intruders. On a couple of occasions they saw a cat disappearing over the back fence, no doubt unnerved by their frequent appearances.

After a week they no longer saw the cat and Snow stopped spraying as he was a lot more relaxed. Snow just needed his frustration and anguish acknowledged, not scolded. The household went back to the harmony it once had, and I was thrilled to have been a successful intermediary.

With communication, patience, consistent training and providing what our beloved animals need for their well-being, you can achieve so much. You can only do this if you are flexible. These beautiful creatures require space to be themselves, whatever species they are. You need to understand their needs as much as you expect them to understand yours. Let's face it, there is nothing more wonderful than sharing our lives with happy, fulfilled animals.

30

Moving House

I HAVE MOVED SEVERAL TIMES WITH MATTIE AND SHEA AND FOUND a few successful methods to keep the stress for them to a minimum. Shea is fairly laid-back, but Mattie is extremely sensitive to anything new, always needing to be certain of her surroundings before she feels comfortable. She feels anxious in any new situation and requires reassurance.

Several days prior or during the most disruptive period of a move you might consider putting flower or gem essences that help with dealing with change in their water bowl. In Bach flower essences you can use rescue remedy and walnut; with Australian bush flower essences, emergency remedy. Continue using it for a week or two after you are in the new premises.

If you have access to the new home prior to the move, take your animals (especially cats) over to that place for a few hours and allow them to familiarise themselves with the new surroundings. By this I mean allowing your cats to be *inside* only, and perhaps inside and outside for dogs, making absolutely sure they aren't able to leave the area. This way they'll become more familiar with the smells and the set up of the new conditions before the big move. The new place will not be foreign to them when you do make the move. I'd do this at least once, hopefully twice, before the actual relocation.

When we do this, Mattie and Shea would be in the cat carrier for at least ten minutes after we arrive at a new home, and they'd meow loud and long. Then, once venturing out, they would proceed with absolute caution, as though there were minefields all over the house, meowing to make us aware they aren't too happy about this. Thankfully they usually only do this on the first visit. By going through this process, it makes our moves relatively anxiety free and the settling in almost immediate.

I suggested these methods to Carmen whose Siamese, Julius, did not want to move and lose the freedom he had to roam (see Chapter 22, 'New Environments'). Carmen said she'd let me know how the move went as far as Julius was concerned. Three weeks later Carmen gave me the update. She couldn't believe how easily Julius had settled in. The suggestions worked, and Julius looked calm and relatively stress free. Julius had not yet ventured out the front of the property near the busy road, and for Carmen that would always be a concern. There will more than likely come a day when he'd find it necessary to explore that area, because he needs to be able to have a sense of his own independence.

Sometimes there are other complicating factors in a move, such as the break-up in a relationship or marriage, with everything haggled over, including your beloved companions. This is debilitating for the people concerned, as well as for your animals who will be torn between the two people they love. There is more often than not extreme tension leading up to a relationship breakdown, and the tension usually continues for some time afterwards, and this can be quite unsettling.

Animals rarely have any say about who they end up with after a split, and they may not see one of their loved persons ever again. It can be very trying, so you'll need to give them much affection, understanding and patience. Just as you need time to heal, so do your animals.

Rory and Elaine were married for five years when they decided to separate. They dearly loved Prince their Golden Retriever but Elaine felt it was better for Prince to reside with her as Rory was often travelling with his work. Elaine was also moving back to the country with her parents and Prince would have lots of room to run around in his new home. With work commitments and Prince being so far away from the city, visits from Rory would be rare. Rory felt devastated. Although Prince loved Elaine it took him several months to adjust to the new living conditions, and the long gaps of time between visits from Rory.

On a brighter note, some animals couldn't be happier about new living conditions. There are times when home actually improves, especially when moving from a confined situation to having a backyard, or being able to roam in bushland. In many instances the reason people instigate this relocation is to provide a better home for their animal companions.

One of the things I love most about animals is that even when they are going through stress, they manage to be there for us as support, offering endless love. All they want for us is love and happiness, so remember to offer this to them also. Animals share such a big part of our lives and we can impact on them so deeply by our actions.

PART V

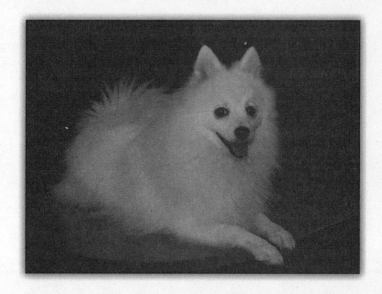

Breeders and Pet Shops

31

Addition to the Family

I AM OFTEN ASKED HOW I FEEL ABOUT BREEDERS AND PET SHOPS. IT'S HARD to figure out where to start on this topic, as there are pros and cons. I *do* know there are already so many animals in the world needing homes, and it is irresponsible for all concerned to breed and sell animals without this being taken into account.

Even in the most extreme circumstances, when we may be forced to give up our animal companions, it's our responsibility to find a safe, suitable and loving home for them. Your animals ending up in an animal refuge should be the last resort. In cases of neglect and abandonment, I have rarely found an excuse for this *inhuman* behaviour. I've heard directly from the animals the effect it has on the rest of their lives should they make it that far. Many end up on death row, and I can assure you they understand they've been abandoned. Can you imagine their sorrow?

As far as breeders go: plenty of families responsibly research the type of animal they wish to have join their family; they do not buy impulsively from a pet shop while out shopping one day—so three cheers for them. Bringing an animal into your life is something that needs a great deal of thought. Which one will suit the home and environment you offer? If you already have animals at home, you'll need to decide if the new one will fit in or, maybe, cause a major disruption. Unfortunately when you see an adorable puppy or kitten looking at you with big brown eyes it's not those considerations that fill your mind. People tend to forget these little cuties grow up and there are responsibilities.

Displaying and selling animals in pet shops is quite a different matter. I find it disturbing when I pass pet shops and hear the words, *Help me, help me*, coming from the birds in those crowded enclosures at the back of the shop.

I wanted to know what the animals in these shops thought about being there, and what it was really like from their perspective. I decided to do some research and went to several pet shops to communicate. There were animals in them that thought it fun playing with the other animals, and being held and played with by different people; and I found that most staff who worked at the pet shops I visited were committed to the wellbeing of the animals. There were a few shops, however, where the animals let me know that at night when the shop was shut they were very frightened of being alone and of hearing strange noises. I couldn't believe these animals were left by themselves overnight.

I decided to literally step into a few of these small animals with my acute sensing, and experience what they were feeling. This is what one young puppy felt:

It was lovely playing with my brother and sister in the enclosure without a care in the world. Then I saw that nice lady approaching with bowls of food and fresh water. As she opened the enclosure we all ran to meet her. She put the bowls down for us and we scrambled to get the food first. She gave us a pat and then closed the door again.

After a big feed we all got very tired and curled up with each other and went to sleep. Then another lady came and opened the enclosure door and she lifted my brother and me out. It was fun being cuddled, then after a short while I was put back with my sister. I waited and waited for my brother, but he never came back. I looked over and saw these people still holding him, and then they walked past us and kept going. I called out to him but he didn't hear.

I wanted to know where they were taking him and whether they'd bring him back.

That same nice lady brought more food and water for us. She gave us another pat and then closed the door. Things were very quiet and then it went dark. So we ate our meal and curled up with each other and went to sleep. I woke up a few times to strange noises but it was still very dark. I could hear barking and crying from other puppies next to us and below us. It was hard to stay asleep. I wished so hard that our mum was here.

After what seemed like an eternity, I heard some more noises and suddenly the place was all lit up again. A girl came over to lift us out and we played for a while on the ground, running around these big packets and toys. Then we were put back in our enclosure. I wish we could stay out and play, even if just for a little bit longer. The enclosure was very clean now and she brought us more food and water.

A lot of people started to come in and look right at us through the glass. I was more interested in playing with my sister, as she's delightful. We became tired and had another sleep. I heard the click of the enclosure door and then my sister was lifted out. I was very concerned as I wanted her to come back. I waited and waited and then she was put back in with me. We curled up again and went to sleep.

It seemed like a long time later when the enclosure was opened again and we ran to meet that nice lady. She always played with us and gave us a pat. But she had only come for my sister. I waited and waited, but this time she didn't return. I just sat there looking through the glass at this little girl holding her and then playing with her on the ground. Then a lady picked up my sister and some parcels and walked away with her.

Now I felt very sad as I was left alone. I wondered where were they taken and what would happen to them. I wondered if I would always be alone in this glass confinement, or would I be taken somewhere? Where? What would become of me?

I stepped out of that puppy's existence with a new understanding of what it felt like for them. Their whole future rested on a person's decision. Perhaps this is what it's like for children in an orphanage, the same thoughts and feelings surging through their minds.

32

Impulse Buying

I DON'T FEEL PET SHOPS ARE THE CORRECT WAY TO FIND THE precious animal to become part of your family. There are so many homeless animals in shelters who badly need a home. Beautiful animals who, due to various circumstances, have found themselves wanting love and a new home.

If you are, however, going to choose a breeder then taking the time to find a reputable one is the only way to go. Those who have a sincere interest in the breed and often show their animals are the ones I'm referring to. They have minimal litters and selectively choose the homes for their babies.

There are, alas, breeders who run animal factories, and I give them a huge thumbs down. It's a money-making business for them and many of their animals are overbred and never see the light of day. They're kept in holding pens and are continually pregnant or feeding offspring. They give birth, nurture their babies for a short time, and then see them taken away without explanation. Then when they're no longer useful they're given away, sold, or end up on death row. The poor things are usually kept in appalling conditions.

The breeding of animals needs to have stricter regulations and there should be a limit on the number of litters an animal can have in one year. There are already thousands of homeless animals without our creating thousands more unnecessarily.

There are also breeds being developed that are definitely not beneficial to the animals. Vets tell me that, with some of the 'designer dogs' around, there's more evidence of hip dysplasia. This is just one particular condition, but there are plenty of others.

By the way, when I refer to 'designer' I mean combining breeds to create a more desirable-looking dog, or one that fits in better with a home environment—such as those who don't shed their hair. When walking along the street one day a man approached me with a dog, the likes of which I had never seen before. It was similar to a Dachshund or 'sausage' dog, but with legs like a Komodo dragon lizard, angled out to the sides. I asked him what type of dog it was and the man said he didn't know. He'd bought it on impulse from a pet shop and told me how difficult it was for the dog to run. Apparently it had already had several visits to the vet regarding his joints.

Was this just a freak of nature—or careless breeding? Did the pet shop concerned only deal with reputable breeders? The responsibility lies with many organisations in any city. People also need to realise that when you invite an animal to join you and your family, there are certain responsibilities attached.

When the hair starts to shed or robust puppies chew everything in sight, or when you want to go on vacation and don't wish to pay for boarding, it's just plain cruel and cowardly to dump these animals or give them to animal refuges. For some people, animals become an inconvenience, and that's why it's so important to give a great deal of thought to these decisions before you bring one into your home. This is an animal's life you're dealing with, and it needs to be taken seriously.

They're relying on you!

33

An Untimely Farewell

THERE IS NO GREATER JOY THAN WELCOMING AN ANIMAL INTO your home, but there are heaps of considerations in the process. For starters, you need to be able to provide all the necessary physical requirements—quality natural nutrition, filtered water where possible, adequate veterinary care if the need should arise, and a suitable safe environment—for the type of animal you choose. Different animals have different requirements.

Animals also don't pack up and move out at a certain age like young adults do. In most cases we watch them go from being babies to toddlers through to adulthood, and finally into old age. Each stage of their lives happens while they live with you, and under your influence. It's a responsibility, but also very much a joy.

Even if you get an animal as an adult, they will still be there with you until their time to leave comes, and the decisions you make for them can be both joyous or catastrophic—so they need to be considered carefully.

In my practice I've had thousands of animals express their delight at being part of a happy family. They tell me they like nothing more than being included in all the events that happen within these homes. They see babies arrive in the house and watch them grow from toddlers into teenagers and beyond, depending on when the animal joined the family, and they feel sad when a child leaves the nest as they may not see as much of them after that. They have also told me about being in their elder years and sharing the corresponding stage of life with their human counterparts.

The impact of the highs and lows felt by the humans of the family is also felt by the animal family. They take you and the events that occur to heart, and want only pleasure and contentment for all concerned. Certain circumstances may come up, like needing to move interstate or overseas, the arrival of a new baby, shifting into an apartment after having a house—the list goes on—and it can cause the family great disruption.

One of these disruptions involves deciding what to do with beloved cats and dogs that may no longer fit into a new lifestyle. At times people feel they have no choice but to find an alternative living arrangement for their animal. This is difficult to discuss, as I know it's very painful for both animals and people to contemplate the great loss this entails—and sometimes the guilt never quite goes away for a family.

Humans in this predicament might look to their friends and family for assistance in finding their precious animal friend a good home. They may even advertise in the newspaper. Either way, in most cases a suitable alternative can be found where the animal can happily live out its days.

In these circumstances, the animal is losing their home and family, and facing a life of uncertainty. All of a sudden in a strange place with unfamiliar faces surrounding them. There may be other animals there already, with whom they may or may not get on, plus their routine and activities can change greatly. Things they enjoyed doing, and the humans they did them with, are now just a memory. They may never see their family members again, and they haven't had anything explained to them—they're just thrust into this new situation.

Imagine how that would feel if it happened to you! Could *you* deal with that?

The worst scenario of course is when the people don't go to that much trouble, choosing instead to surrender their animals to a pound. This is a devastating choice, even though there are many staff at these organisations who love animals. The reality is that these animals are placed in an enclosure, the food is different, and there are all these other animals, and nothing but uncertainty about what lies ahead.

I communicated with a dog called Samuel after he had been put down, and he gave me his heart-wrenching account of being in this very situation. Sam, as he was affectionately known, was a cream-coloured Maltese cross. He had had his paws up against a glass enclosure of the local pet shop when Hillary and her two-year-old twin sons, Jamie and Josh, first set eyes on him, standing there as cute as a button with his soft wavy fur and big brown eyes. Only eight weeks old, but full of energy and enthusiasm.

Hillary hadn't intended on having a pet at this stage, as life was busy enough with two small children. However, when she saw him in the window she simply had to go in. The two boys were begging her, 'Puppy, Mummy, puppy.' She couldn't resist them and asked the attendant if she could hold Sam.

As he was placed in her arms, there was a sense of her heart melting with love. We have all experienced this feeling at some stage with an adorable baby animal. And when Jamie and Josh's eyes lit up as they were allowed to stroke the puppy, Hillary's mind was made up . . . this puppy was going home with them.

Unfortunately, when she got home, Sam was not met by the same warm, fuzzy feeling from Hillary's husband, Robert. He was extremely annoyed that this decision had been made without him, but as time went by, things settled down and Sam became a part of this merry gang.

He loved being around people and other animals and was always eager to please. The two young boys adored him, and Hillary always made an effort to take him for a walk and to play with him. He went on family outings and was crazy about the excitement of the boys' birthdays. He loved the ripping of paper from the presents and the joy on Jamie's and Josh's faces as the surprise was revealed. After being with the family for nine years he certainly got to see many birthdays.

Sam was a dog who liked nothing better than having fun and sharing that fun with people. He'd do anything to make Hillary, Robert and the boys smile. He'd perform tricks to make them laugh and then run in circles around the children to get them to play.

Then one day came the news that shattered Sam's dream world. Robert announced to Hillary that, as a company director, he was being sent overseas indefinitely. They needed to be relocated within a month.

Hillary didn't fully comprehend at that point what was to come. The next couple of weeks were bedlam, with boxes being packed and people coming and going. Sam was very confused about was happening in his normally serene world.

Robert then asked Hillary what she would do with the dog. Hillary naturally assumed he'd join them. Robert told her that this was out of the question, as initially they'd be living in an apartment until they found a suitable residence. Added to that, quarantine would be too difficult and expensive. There were many arguments until Robert finally got his way. Hillary then frantically rang around friends and relatives to see if anyone could take him.

With no success, she resorted to an advert in the newspaper—but only one call resulted, and it wasn't tempting. Hillary was devastated. After all, she cared for Sam almost as much as she did her children, and had never considered giving him up.

Feeling anxious, Hillary explained to Robert that although trying as hard as she could, she hadn't yet found a suitable home for Sam. With only a week to go before they flew out, Robert felt there was no alternative but to take Sam to the pound.

When the awful day arrived, Hillary couldn't bring herself to go along. She cried non-stop all morning.

Sam remembers it so clearly. He and his bed were bundled into the car, with Robert silent through the journey. When they arrived at the pound Robert went in first and left Sam in the car. Then he came out and got Sam and his bed. He handed them over to this lady and Sam watched as Robert left without even turning back.

Sam was totally bewildered as to why he was in this strange place. At first he thought he may just be there for a bit, while there were so many things going on at home. Iris, the lady at the pound, gave him a cuddle and then put him and his bed into a cage which had a cold floor, and he was locked in. He sat there for a while looking around and could see many other dogs in cages barking and whimpering. He was hoping like heck that he didn't have to stay too long and that he could soon go home. Days passed and many people wandered through to view the dogs. Sam would run up to the front of the cage and look for his family—but all in vain. Each day he thought this would be the day they came to collect him. As the attendants brought him out to be inspected by visitors, he felt quiet and withdrawn and would then run to the back of his enclosure. It wasn't that he didn't like people, but he was waiting for his family. He was sure they would come, and of course this attitude didn't make him very appealing to anyone wanting a friendly dog!

While many of the other dogs found homes, unfortunately for Sam, he didn't. As time went on, the penny dropped for Sam that maybe they weren't going to come for him. He wondered how this could be, because he loved them and they loved him. Why would they forget about him? Why would they leave him in this strange place? What would become of him now?

He became increasingly withdrawn and depressed. And his only salvation was Iris, who'd come to sit and chat to him, or take him outside for fresh air. But this still didn't fill the void of losing his loved ones. Sam so missed the laughter of the children.

Weeks turned into months and it was unlikely Sam would ever be placed in a new home. With limited space at the shelter there was no alternative but death row. Once there, he was allowed just another six weeks in which to find a placement. Unfortunately his time was slowly running out.

One night Iris and another attendant came to get Sam out of the enclosure and take him to a different part of the pound—to a room he recalled being in before when a vet had checked him on his first day there. Iris was holding him and stroking him. She began whispering, 'Everything will be all right,' and tears filled her eyes. Sam could feel her extreme sadness and wanted to help.

Iris placed Sam in his bed on the stainless steel table, still stroking him and reassuring him. Just then, another attendant pulled out his paw and he felt the prick of a needle and a sudden coldness travel up his leg. He began to feel a weariness come over him, he couldn't keep his eyes open. Although trying to fight this tiredness, Sam succumbed and as he closed his eyes he slowly looked up at Iris. Within seconds he lay limp in her arms and he was gone, finally at peace.

Many people don't understand what it's like from an animal's point of view when they're abandoned—whether they will be lucky enough to find another home where there will be love and someone to take care of them or whether their luck will run out . . . just as Sam's did.

PART VI

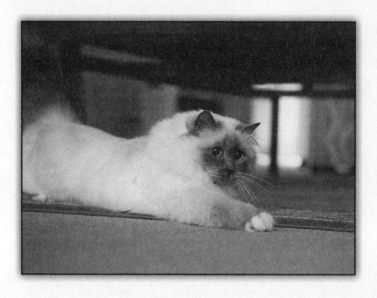

Competitive Arenas

34

The Horses that Didn't Want to Race

THERE ARE MANY ANIMALS BRED FOR RACING, BUT LET'S LOOK at horses. The sport of kings, as it's known, is a source of pleasure (and sometimes despair!) for billions of people around the world, but horseracing can be a cruel business. I want to discuss what it's like for horses that race, or are in other competitive arenas. There's so much money put into these horses to win that if they don't perform they're not financially viable. It's as simple and brutal as that.

Horses are a very large animal so all the things associated with keeping a horse are expensive. Just for starters, you have vet bills, feed costs, the housing of such a large animal and the provision of a sizable place for it to roam. With performing horses, add in trainers, jockeys, specialised vets, equipment, and the time spent to prepare them for races.

Even if you invest in the best facilities and equipment it doesn't ensure a horse will do well, just as it doesn't guarantee it for an athlete. Many try, but don't succeed. Unfortunately for horses, if they don't succeed, they end up being shuffled around from owner to owner or, at the worst, it's off to the knackery with them.

The X-factor, which isn't usually looked at in these situations, is the passion to win. Many horses simply don't want to race or jump or event. These activities have been *chosen* for them. You often hear of people complaining that when they were young they were made to do hours of practice a day on a musical instrument they despised or in a sport they hated. They would much rather have been having fun playing games with their friends. There are many reasons for an animal's discontent. The ones I have found among the most common are boredom, confinement, lack of choices, performance anxiety, an incorrect bit or saddle, and back injury or soreness.

Juniper was a deep-brown thoroughbred regarded by those around him as having unlimited potential. He had won a race once and drawn places at other times. When his part-owner, Craig, contacted me he wasn't even drawing places. Craig felt Juniper was down about something but he couldn't figure out what. Once I had communicated with Juniper, it all came to light.

Being highly intelligent, he was able to tell me that he was bored and wanted more variety in his training. He made it clear that he was normally a very enthusiastic, energetic horse—and that this lack of stimulation was getting him down. Every day seemed the same to him, with rarely a break from routine. He also told me that his hind back area was very sore. When ridden, the saddle was causing pressure on these tender areas and this was also discouraging him from training.

I discussed the actual races with Juniper to see if anything could be improved and discovered he didn't like being in the middle of the pack on race day, as it made him feel confined. He preferred to come through on the outside where he felt freer and more relaxed.

Craig took all this information on board and began to make some changes. He made training more stimulating and varied. He had Juniper's back checked and they found a malalignment which they began treating. Craig had his saddle modified to make it more comfortable in that area of Juniper's back. He also informed the jockey about taking him to the outside when racing.

Juniper was thrilled at having his needs acknowledged, and his racing started to come together. Slowly, he began to place again and even took a few wins within the first few months. Craig commented that he could see Juniper was running with passion once more.

There's that magic word again: passion!

Sadly, running with passion wasn't the case for Caddy who had lost love of racing. His new trainer, Lucy, was concerned as Caddy was very down and quite often aggressive. His owners wanted him performing as soon as possible, but first Lucy wanted to know how he felt about racing.

I settled down for a chat with Caddy and soon found out that he literally hated it, showing me upsetting images of how he'd been punished with a whip when he hadn't performed. Everything was so strict and routine, with no room for fun. Caddy felt he'd been moved around from place to place and was never able to establish relationships with horses or humans. The only humans he had contact with didn't care about him as an individual, and were preoccupied only with how he raced. I could sense he really needed to be loved (don't we all!). He was a horse that was quite driven emotionally, and this needed to be addressed. Caddy told me he just wanted to be in a field of grass, grazing as horses were meant to. He just longed to be a horse in its true sense.

I explained to Lucy that I didn't feel confident that she could conquer this particular equine mindset about racing, because Caddy had had enough and wanted to retire. Lucy's fear was that the owners had told her that if she didn't lift him up to racing standard, he'd go to the knackery. She had grown very fond of Caddy and decided if he didn't end up racing well, she'd buy him herself to ensure his safety.

These cases are as individual as the horses are. Achieving this understanding of how they feel, or the changes they need, can greatly change outcomes. If your heart is not in something it's very hard to succeed.

However, a change of heart is very possible.

35

On Show

A STORY I SIMPLY MUST TELL IS ABOUT MR RED, A HORSE WITH amazing confidence and knowledge. He was a renowned racehorse who, lately, hadn't been making the winning circle as often as before. His owner, Miranda, adored this horse, and their relationship was like mother and son.

Miranda knew Mr Red wished he could do well again, and she wanted to help him achieve his goal, as any mother would. When I talked with Mr Red, boy was he confident. Right off the bat I asked if he liked racing, and he replied that what he really loved was the adulation of the crowd after a win . . . the way the crowd rose to their feet in sheer excitement. But more importantly, he treasured the adulation of Miranda. He worshiped her.

Mr Red also said to me that he liked to show the other horses on the racetrack who was boss. So I asked if there was a reason he wasn't quite making the wins so often any more. He let me know he wasn't surprised that winning was eluding him. He felt the jockeys were morons. Mr Red certainly didn't mince words!

I asked him to explain what he meant and he replied that he was the horse, and *he* was the one doing the running. He wanted a jockey who would let him run his own race.

I wondered if he had one in mind. Mr Red said, *There's one jockey who rides light (*by 'light' he meant riding in a less-restraining manner*).*

I spoke with Miranda and she knew instantly who that jockey was. So we gave the jockey in question instructions to allow Mr Red plenty of leeway to run his own race. I also asked Miranda to allow the jockey to visit Mr Red the day before the race, so Mr Red would know which jockey would be riding him in the race the next day. The jockey agreed with our requests and Mr Red easily beat the field. Miranda couldn't believe the way he was strutting around afterwards. He was really playing to the crowd.

Mr Red wasn't the only one to prance around with self-assurance. This was also true of Priscilla, an amazing white thoroughbred. And I have to say that when I first set eyes on her she took my breath away with her beauty. She was the type of horse I dreamt about when I was a child.

Priscilla was a dressage horse and her carer was Katrina who had ridden her in competition for many years. Now Katrina was concerned that Priscilla, although extremely fit, was getting to an age where she may prefer to be retired. She adored Priscilla and wanted what was best for her, which was music to my ears!

Communicating with Priscilla soon answered that question. She told me she definitely didn't want to retire, as she still got a buzz from hearing the comments of various people on competition day who admired her beauty and her abilities. Priscilla felt if she didn't train and compete she'd be bored and wasting her talents. She, like Mr Red, certainly didn't suffer from a lack of confidence.

It is not only horses who love to parade and show off, and my mind now turns to an amazing caramel Saluki dog named Rafik. His owner was my friend, Max, who idolised Rafik—Rafik was certainly difficult to take your eyes off. Salukis are a very sleek dog with the most graceful movements. It was no wonder Max wanted to show him off, but unfortunately Rafik was interested one minute, and disinterested the next.

Communicating with Rafik was always a rewarding experience, as this was a dog that didn't hold back. He was happy to tell me the whole story, describing how he loved to throw his head high and show himself to the public in the way that he felt best displayed his characteristics. This of course didn't always conform to the rules of showing. Rafik was extremely intelligent and quite hyperactive, so this combination did not suit the quieter times in between dog show events. He found these lulls in the proceedings extremely boring, and he couldn't understand why the show had to take all day.

His only regret was that he felt he was letting Max down. Rafik knew how much Max wanted to be at these shows. He loved Max and didn't want to disappoint him.

As it turned out, Max's reaction was that he didn't want to make Rafik do the dog shows under sufferance. He wanted to do things with Rafik that they both enjoyed, and he soon found that a run along the beach was an activity they were both enthusiastic about. And I'm pleased to report they continue to make this their regular pastime.

These success stories always seem to go hand-in-hand with love and respect. And when you really think about it, that isn't too much to ask, is it?

36

When Animals Vanish

THE DISAPPEARANCE OF YOUR ANIMAL IS A DEVASTATING experience. Even with the best intentions, accidents can happen—you thought the lawnmower man closed the gate or that the kids had closed the front door. Initially you panic with an urgency and desperation to find them as soon as possible. Every minute that goes by is another minute your loved one is out there and facing the elements. It is like a ticking time bomb in your head. You want them back safely, because they're family members, like one of your own children.

This opens up many questions in people's minds. Are they safe? Have they been picked up by someone? Will that person keep them, or hand them in? Have they been run over? Has anything awful happened to them? Can they find their own way home? Will I ever see them again? Are they hungry? It's so cold . . . what if they can't find any shelter? Are they terrified? Will they think I'm not looking for them?

You can't seem to stop these questions continually rushing through your head. You wished you had put an identification tag on your beloved friend. You were going to, but hadn't quite got round to it. There is a sense of guilt. Indeed, there can be a lot of guilt associated with a lost animal. It also generates a feeling of hopelessness when you fail to find them after a period of time. People feel they have let their animals down by not protecting them. Because of this, it's not surprising that many people turn to an animal communicator for assistance.

I've discovered that certain animal communicators choose not to do this type of work—as it can be much more difficult than the usual communication work and doesn't always have a happy ending. I have to admit it's not the easiest part of my work, and it was very daunting when I first started out. There is a lot of pressure, which doesn't help the situation, and you need to remain very calm and focused for the connection with the animal. The pressure firstly is the urgency, and the feeling of fear and hopelessness from the person for the safety of their much-loved animal family member. Secondly, I worry about my abilities to gain the details needed to find this animal. There's always my own sense of desperation in wanting to find this lost animal quickly.

It's often like finding a needle in a haystack, as the animal may be frightened or disorientated. If they've run off chasing another animal, are being chased themselves, or are following a scent, then their preoccupation with this allows them to miss the details of their trail.

It's possible to get a sense of whether the animal is alive or not, or if the animal intends returning home within a certain timeframe. Tuning into the animal can help in assessing their emotional and physical state. It can determine if the animal is alone, with people or another animal.

This situation can be absolutely terrifying for an animal, especially if they have never been away from home before. They may be coming into contact with other animals, strange people and vehicles. Each animal will act differently in these predicaments. Some will run and hide for protection and others will be more trusting and willingly approach a stranger. This stranger could be the help needed to find the animal, as they may take the animal to their local vet or pound, so contacting the vets, pounds and animal shelters in your area should be your first priority.

Unfortunately, approaching strangers can also be an animal's downfall, should that person choose to keep the animal for themselves or choose to torment or cause them harm.

Some animals will also choose to confront another animal rather than run, which could lead to an injury. As you can see there are so many scenarios.

When trying to locate lost animals I try to tune into the animal on my own in a quiet place so there are no distractions. Some animals, using visualisation, are able to show me the direction from which they left their home, and their journey to where they are at present. This greatly assists in locating them. There are also tools that I use on occasions such as a pendulum. A pendulum is an intuitive tool that can enable you to access or confirm a direction by its swing. These were used in ancient times to answer many questions and are still used frequently today.

Remote viewing is also an intuitive tool, and is imagining looking through the eyes of that particular animal and at its surroundings. This is definitely an art, and the information subjective, so it can at times be disappointing, as an exact location is difficult to pinpoint. However, using this technique has enabled landmarks to be picked up, which can be identified by the animal's owner. You must remember many lost animals are frightened and hungry so are often preoccupied with survival.

The information can also vary from moment to moment. Animals, unless asleep or injured, can be on the move, so the details might be quite different with each connection I have with them. Asking them to stay still can be difficult as they need to hunt for food, water and shelter and won't stop until that is accomplished. Their current surroundings may also be unsafe, so the need to move on can be urgent.

After a few days of being lost, animals tend to revert to their instinctual nature to survive in these outside circumstances. That is why some cats have returned to their wild instincts: what we humans refer to as feral. They may not even respond to their name when you call out, due to the fear of people approaching—whether they know them or not.

There are many reasons that make it difficult to guarantee success. On many occasions animals have been located. Owners whose animals haven't been found, although heartbroken, can still find a degree of closure when they know they have tried every avenue to find them. When you love someone deeply, you don't want to give up. You try every possibility, until all are exhausted.

Nadine, due to circumstances beyond her control, had to live overseas for a time, leaving her beloved horse, Monty, with a close friend, Mandy. As far as she knew, everything was okay for Monty. Upon her return, she intended to resettle him with her. But when she came back, to her horror, she found a very different story: Monty was no longer with Mandy!

Mandy confessed sheepishly that it had proved impossible to keep him, and so she'd placed him temporarily with a friend of hers. Nadine couldn't believe what Mandy was telling her. Then things went from bad to worse, with Mandy admitting this person had since put Monty up for auction!

Nadine was devastated, unable to understand how and why Mandy could have done what she did. And no matter how many times she asked, Mandy avoided the question. Then after exhaustive inquiries, Nadine eventually found out the address of Mandy's friend, and this woman simply said she had no idea where Monty was now. Nadine spent months pestering staff at the auction centre and tracing records, but Monty seemed to have vanished into thin air.

When she came to see me she needed some answers and was hoping I could help her. She loved her horse so much and was finding his loss difficult to bear.

I connected with Monty, instantly sensing a very light and distant presence. I asked him if he was deceased and he said, *Yes*. I then inquired if he could give me details of what had happened to him after the auction, telling him that Nadine was suffering from terrible guilt as she felt she'd let him down.

Monty asked me to tell Nadine not to feel this way as he understood that she couldn't help what had happened. He loved her deeply and looked forward to when they would be one day reunited. It was a good outcome.

Monty showed me the day at the auction and how he was taken by a couple who had showjumping horses. He said they thought he'd be suitable, but when things didn't work out, he ended up back at the auction arena. Then a man bought him who owned a cattle farm and wanted Monty as a workhorse. Monty said the work was very hard, pulling heavy things. But he was kept apart from the other horses and fed the barest amount of hay. Monty had been so lonely, so unhappy.

Monty went on to tell me that one day he injured his leg, and he knew that once he was lame he'd no longer be any good to the farmer. He remembers the vet coming out and examining his leg, shaking his head and saying, 'This is a bad injury, and it will be expensive and time-consuming to repair. There are no guarantees of full recovery.'

Monty heard the farmer replying, 'It's time to get rid of him.' Monty said he wasn't quite sure what he meant, but knew he'd have no choice in the decision.

A few minutes later the vet approached him and next thing he felt the coldness of a needle going into his body. This made him very drowsy. Monty felt he needed to lie down, and when he did he remembers the vet coming over to him again and then he lost consciousness. Drifting high above in the clouds, he noticed how light he felt and began soaring high and higher. He felt free. Free.

I was feeling incredibly emotional at hearing all of this, but I knew I had to find out if there was anything Monty wished to say to Nadine. He said, *Tell her not to grieve for me, as I am in a beautiful place where the freedom of my soul is able to roam. Grief will tie her down and restrict her journey. I will watch over her and walk beside her on her journey.*

It was difficult for me to discuss the details of his death with Nadine but, although heartbroken, she said, 'At least I can stop frantically looking for him, constantly coming up against deadends in my search.' She soulfully remarked that at least now she had closure—best of all, that she now knew he was free.

37

Where Do Animals Go When They Die?

WHEN YOUR BELOVED ANIMAL PASSES AWAY IT CAN BE DEVASTATING, especially given it tends to leave many unanswered questions. Where do they go? Who is with them? Are they okay? And plenty of people are keen to know if their darling, departed companion has a soul.

Human anxiety about death seems to be a combination of fear of the unknown, fear of experiencing great suffering and pain during the dying process, and/or fear of dying alone. We're inclined to imagine that our animals experience the same concerns, and this can contribute to the extreme distress we may go through in making euthanasia decisions. But, interestingly, while most people imagine that animals are going through those same fears as *we* do, it's not the case.

I have to admit that before I became an animal communicator my mindset about death was similar to what I've described here. Sure, we're all going to pass over at some stage, but it isn't what you want to think about.

I now have a different perception, as animals have shown me a new way of looking at death and dying. Thanks to them, I'm now in a place that allows me to regard death as not being as scary and final as I had once thought. Or to put it another way: they've taught me that dying is just one of many experiences we all go through.

Animals have said to me that people need to live life in the moment. Yes, the goal is to make the most of our time on earth but, at the same time, it's also about creating the person we wish to become.

PART VII

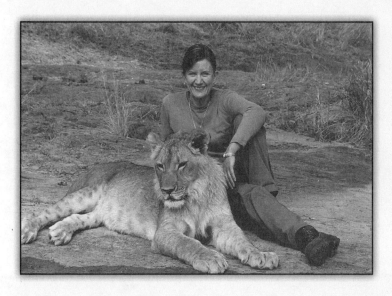

Respecting the
Natural World

38

What Cats Have to Say

MOST WOMEN CAN'T RESIST A GORGEOUS CAT; FOR SOME REASON females and felines are a great combination. Sure, plenty of men have cats, but the mutual attraction isn't quite so strong. And perhaps that's because cats resemble women with their complex personalities and at times, unpredictability. I have found felines to be one of the most intuitive species of all animals, and that's a big part of their pulling power for me.

Cats live totally in the moment and can be observed in their own little world, appearing to be completely oblivious of what's happened around them. They have this uncanny way of letting us know that they are otherwise engaged, which at first appears antisocial. But they're actually showing us how to live our lives to the full. It matters not what is in our past, as that is over and done with, and has nothing to do with our future—who knows if and what will occur.

Cats, wise creatures that they are, understand that all we have control over is the present, and they're utterly preoccupied with making the most out of what is right now. Live every moment and fill them with the things that make your heart sing. This is what they're saying to us, which is incredible food for the soul, isn't it?

Cats love to play, even into old age, and they make *us* feel like we're never too old for fun. When cats play it's simplistic, and this teaches us how to enjoy what's already around us. They'll make a game out of literally anything, like the washing when you're trying to fold it. I might be attempting to put plastic containers away into the cupboard and they'll treat that as a game too, kicking bits of Tupperware around the kitchen floor. There's no stopping them! Felines find this sort of nonsense highly amusing, and they seem to think we do as well.

Not having children of my own means that the birthdays of my 'fur kids' are very important in our household. I set off to the shops to buy something special for Mattie or Shea, our wonderful Birman cats, always managing to come home with an intricate device with a manufacturer's promise of hours of enjoyment for your cats. I remember one year purchasing a transparent jar with a rounded bottom that rocked from side to side when pushed. When you turned the switch on, air was generated inside the jar, which caused paper butterflies to fly around furiously. I thought this was a winner for sure. I had the camera on, ready to capture their initial excitement.

Mattie and Shea slowly approached the unknown object. While Shea looked on intently, Mattie, the girl with the curious heart, gave a gentle nudge with her paw. The jar began to rock, back and forth and then stop. I turned on the switch and watched as the paper butterflies took flight.

Both cats stood to attention, but after a few seconds they walked away, disinterested. I couldn't believe it—my present was boring!

I didn't give up though, and I enticed the two of them back a few times, thinking perhaps they needed to watch a little longer in order to create the excitement I was looking for. Unfortunately the only one in the room the butterflies excited was me! It was quite disheartening.

A few minutes later they were playing fast and furious in the lounge. Leaping high into the air and chasing each other. There appeared to be something in Mattie's mouth, so I went to investigate. It was a shoe string that had been left lying around. The toy I had bought would never change—it was what it was—whereas the shoestring left so much to their imaginations.

We can easily overlook that it's the simple things which create the greatest pleasure. Take time out to play and engage in laughter with others, and with your animals. Learn to be silly. Learn to be a child again. Learn to use your imagination. You may be surprised at what unfolds.

Relaxation is also something cats do extremely well. They rarely run around, unless playing. Smart things that they are, they'll always take time out for themselves, whether it is sleeping in a comfortable spot, sunning themselves on a window ledge, or sitting quietly, meticulously grooming their paws and coats.

Their movements are more of a stroll or saunter, as though they have all the time in the world at their disposal. I can tell you that they're in a semi-meditative state more often than not, and I must admit I'm envious! It's in this state that you are alerted to your inner self, with the added bonus of a greater awareness of your senses. You will hear, see, and smell things that you were totally oblivious of previously.

Discover what really exists in your world—not just what's in front of your face. Be like a cat: relax, and allow all the stresses to pass you by. Let the biggest decision in your day be what to do next with your time.

Cats tend to be very solitary, and we all know how independent they can be. This is indeed beguiling—although I accept that non-cat lovers are inclined to be irritated by that very independence. Cats certainly need their own space, and they'll let you know about it. And they don't hesitate in being vocal or demonstrative to convey their demands.

I find them endlessly fascinating, especially their ability to live their lives on *their* terms. The fact is they rarely like to be governed by others. Learning to be independent and self-reliant, while maintaining the ability to ask for what you need, are definitely feline traits.

When you live with cats, you have the opportunity to emulate them and discover the perfect balance between making time for yourself and being social when it suits you.

Cats will also share their prey with you. This can be either as a hunter's triumph, when they wish to parade their prowess, or as though you are a kitten and they are taking care of you. They are showing you how important you are to them.

Barry had a gorgeous, sleek, pure black Burmese cat named Apollo. Apollo had a dominant presence about him. Barry was quite distressed at finding dismembered rats and mice on his living-room rug. Previously Apollo brought them only to the back door, and Barry just removed them without a fuss. He felt Apollo had gone too far bringing the dead animals into the house. Barry scolded him and threw the dismembered animal into the bin with disgust. He couldn't believe when it happened again the next day, and again he scolded Apollo. The very next night Apollo brought in a dead python and laid it lifeless in the middle of the prized rug. This was the last straw for Barry and he contacted me.

Apollo saw himself as a great hunter and felt he needed to prove his worth as a provider in the house. These dismembered animals were his grand offerings to Barry. Apollo felt the hard work of his hunt and the amazing skills he was displaying did not deserve to go unnoticed. He felt he should be honoured and praised for his achievement. When that didn't happen, and he was shown such disapproval by Barry, he felt his offerings needed to be far bolder and more courageous. The python was actually a predator, not just prey. He had killed and displayed the most dangerous of animals in his environment. Apollo couldn't understand why such a prize was not honoured. I explained to Barry that by giving credit to Apollo through simple praise there would be no need for Apollo to keep displaying his prize.

Barry finally understood and felt quite privileged by Apollo's desire for his approval. He began to praise Apollo for his hunting skills and then removed his victims from the rug out to the back of the house, until Apollo finally realised there was no need a need for him to bring them inside. In fact, after a short while, Apollo no longer displayed them at all.

Occasionally the people in our lives are proud of something they've done and want our approval, but they're disregarded like Apollo was. Say a small child is building a creation out of Leggo and is taking great pride in it. Many times this effort will get passed over without recognition. They're told too quickly to put the toys away, and a rather large hand comes down and destroys their masterpiece.

It only takes a few minutes of praise and appreciation to begin building the stairs to confidence in a person's or an animal's life, and even less time to bring it tumbling down.

It's also true that cats spend much of their time snoozing, which is built into their genes. Lions in the wild can sleep around twenty-two of the twenty-four hours in a day; they do this to conserve their energy for the big hunt. Cats know that sleep assists in the preservation, not only of your physical body, but also of your emotional and spiritual self. It's certainly something for us to keep in mind with our busy lives.

It's well known that many of the human illnesses in modern society comes from a lack of rest, and for being over-stressed, whereas cats will always make room for rest, no matter what. This is a great principle to live by.

Have you noticed that some cats sleep with one eye open? That's so they can be ready for danger, or an opportunity. The lesson for us is that if we keep our minds and awareness open to the world at all times, opportunities will come our way. This is why some people seem to get all the good luck, and others very little. In reality, we all get offered a similar number of opportunities. It's just that some people lack observation, or they delay taking action. Meanwhile, cats rarely miss an opportunity.

Our feline friends are confident and usually fearless. Often times I've watched one prepare to take a leap that looks absolutely impossible to me. They'll apply tremendous focus, without giving away the slightest hint of wanting to give up, or of nervousness. With their body poised and a light swaying back and forth of readiness—like a tightrope walker—they're not thinking of how perilous the feat might be. They are totally absorbed in where they want to go or what they want to do. The goal is foremost in their minds, with no time for disbelief or doubt. It's thrilling to watch.

Felines trust their instincts and intuitive senses, and in most cases will succeed with ease and confidence. And even if they don't succeed, they brush themselves off and try again, or move on to another amusement. No big deal. We should look to them for inspiration in our own lives, keeping our eye on the prize.

Humans are inclined to live lives that are filled with fear and regret, but it's better to have tried than to have never followed your heart. We tend to focus on the negatives rather than on the possibility of good outcomes. If we believe we can't, then we won't. Trust in yourself and your abilities. Learn from your cat.

At times we come to loggerheads with our pussy cats and they'll have a tantrum. But moments later they're purring up to us and all is forgiven and forgotten. This is probably one of the most amazing attributes of animals. Imagine if every time *we* had an argument or a harsh word with another person, that things could so easily and speedily moved forward. Forgiveness is one of the hardest things for humans to achieve, because our pride gets in the way.

Don't get me wrong: it's not that cats aren't proud; they just perceive things differently, and they don't have to be right all the time—even though most times they think they are! Cats see things in a calmer perspective, and after a scuffle will move on, more preoccupied with creating love and harmony in not only *our* lives—but within the wider world. They know that by always trying to be right, you run the risk of missing out on golden opportunities.

39

Why Animals Disappear

THERE ARE MANY REASONS AN ANIMAL CAN GO MISSING THAT are beyond our control. A storm is a common reason for many dogs to suddenly disappear from the backyard. They can become really distressed by the electrical energy created by a storm, and by the intensity of noise. They get into a state of panic and run to get away from these disturbances. You may remember your own childhood experiences with storms, perhaps being so terrified that you ran from your own room into the safety and security of your parent's bed. Unfortunately, by the time a storm is over, an animal could have travelled some distance and, because they have been so agitated, they won't have a clue of the distance or the direction they've travelled. They can stay in hiding from fear for several days, which makes them difficult to locate.

There are times when animals can go missing while being minded by a friend or family member. You may have gone away on holiday, or been renovating your home. It's so frustrating when you've taken steps to save your much-loved animals the anguish of unsettling disruption or made sure they were with someone familiar in your absence, and they go missing. These types of situations are sometimes unavoidable.

This is what happened to a beautiful seal point Burmese named Lucia. She went missing while temporarily staying with Marcia's parents, while extensive renovations were done. Marcia took her two Burmese cats, Lucia and Renata, to stay with her mum and dad as she felt the cats would be safer and calmer without all the renovation noises. It sounded like a good plan but one afternoon, when the two cats were sitting together on the front porch, Lucia disappeared.

Before Marcia contacted me she had already been in touch with vets and pounds, distributed flyers in letterboxes and placed posters on various street poles in the surrounding area. But when she hadn't received one single phone call, she became extremely worried.

I was able to communicate with Lucia and she revealed that three school children on bikes had lured her over to them, and had then taken her to their home. Nothing sinister; it just seemed like a good idea to these youngsters, as they wanted to play with Lucia.

Renata told me that Lucia was the more confident of the two, so it's wasn't surprising then that she been the one to stroll over towards the children to investigate. It is often beneficial to also communicate with the other animal involved with the one who has gone missing. Communicating again with Lucia, she showed me a backyard with a shed and wooden slats nearby. I could also hear a dog barking in the vicinity. She showed me two people offering her food, but she was too afraid to take it from them.

I revealed to Marcia that her beloved Lucia was near, perhaps only a few houses away. After I had described the children to Marcia, she immediately thought of a house two doors down, where there were three children. Unfortunately, after talking to their mother, it turned out they didn't have Lucia.

Marcia hadn't put any flyers in the letterboxes across the road as it was a four-laned highway and she didn't think it possible for Lucia to cross it. I disagreed with her, explaining I had a vision of her being carried away from the house, so there was every reason to think Lucia could have made it safely across the busy road. On my advice, Marcia took flyers over there immediately, and within four to five hours received a phone call from a house directly opposite.

Marcia went straight over and saw her beloved Lucia huddled near the back shed up on some wooden slats . . . just as Lucia had communicated the scene to me.

The couple who owned the house said they'd discovered her in the backyard because their German Shepherd wouldn't stop barking at her. When questioning their children, they said that she escaped from them in the backyard and they didn't see which way she went. They then forgot about her. The couple even offered Lucia food but she seemed too afraid to accept it.

Marcia was elated to have found Lucia. It just goes to show, never assume the circumstances as you could be wrong and miss out on recovering your loved one. Always cover the bases.

No matter what the outcome, for most people it's just a relief to know the facts, and be able to have closure. It is the not knowing that is so devastating.

40

The Cat in Need of a New Home

THE MORE COMPLEX REASONS WHY SOME ANIMALS GO MISSING may astound you. I'll bet it never occurred to you that what they're often doing is mirroring *our* lives in this situation.

Think back: there may have been a time in your life when you lost direction and plunged into a state of confusion. Perhaps you were in a job you didn't like, working long hours without satisfaction. Or you may have moved from job to job to job in a few years, not able to find one that suited you or gave you that sense of fulfilment. In your own mind you were not even sure what you wanted to do, or where you wanted to go. Inside that head of yours was nothing but confusion and chaos. Know the feeling?

An animal may leave home to show you that, just like them, you're lost and need to find your way. And furthermore, maybe you're not looking at all the possible avenues to get back on the right path—it's not time to give up, but rather, take action. Just as you'd do if your precious animal went missing.

This is mind-blowing stuff, I realise that, but it's all true. I know, because they've told me. Animals may feel unhappiness in their present situation. Perhaps there's an imbalance in the harmony of their environment. There may be financial stress due to mortgage payments, credit card bills, household expenses, and not knowing how you'll come up with the funds. There may be a volatile situation in your relationship, whether verbal or physical. You might be dealing with unruly teenagers and trying to gain some control, but with little success. Each of these sorts of situations is capable of leading to endless abusive arguments and continuous stress. This can be very debilitating for you and also for the animals are living with you.

All of this negativity has the potential to greatly affect their disposition. Animals love us so deeply that they'll most likely become severely stressed if their humans are experiencing difficulties. If they just cannot stay and witness these horrors any longer, they may well flee in desperation. They're wise enough to know that solving these problems can only be achieved by the people themselves, and they'll often find another home elsewhere, where there is peace and harmony. It does make sense.

They know that in a serene environment, contentment will surround both animals and humans, and a state of health and wellbeing will prevail. There are also those animals that just need time out. They have their own issues and experiences to deal with, just as we do. Some are loners by nature, others prefer to have a quieter environment. Maybe they're craving more one-on-one time with their person, but, lately, he or she is too busy. And often, if there are too many other animals in the house, this can be impossible, driving an animal to leave.

Honestly, you need to be realistic about the number of animals you have in one household, and give consideration to the variation of different species. The requirements of all different species need to be met, not dominated by one particular species or animal. For example, cats cannot roam freely in the backyard if they're fearful of large dogs constantly chasing them. Occasionally they're even ravaged, which is just dreadful.

Many of these occasions go unnoticed by the people in the household and, if it comes to their attention, they may lock the cats inside for their protection. This isn't desirable for cats (if they were outdoor cats previously) as it's a complete loss of liberty, and it can lead to their wanting to find somewhere else to live. This was the situation with Queen, a part-Persian tortoiseshell cat. She had been gone ten days when Paula contacted me.

Paula said that Queen had periodically gone away over the last six months, but had never previously stayed away longer than five or six days. Apparently she was quite an independent feline—although inclined to become anxious in certain circumstances. Queen was not desexed and already had two litters to her credit, with Paula having kept a male kitten from the last litter who was now around six months old. She also had Queen's brother, and had just introduced a Labrador puppy to the household. Quite a mixture I must say, but not uncommon.

I communicated with Queen and she told me she had found herself a temporary second home with a couple a short distance from Paula's place. She liked it there as she was the only animal; it was very peaceful. She described her home with Paula as noisy and disruptive, and she was constantly harassed by the two male cats. The introduction of the puppy was the last straw for her! As our conversation went on, she revealed that she had in fact decided to make her temporary refuge permanent. She also informed me she was in kitten again and didn't want to give birth to her babies amid all the disruptions at Paula's.

I let Paula know what was going on in Queen's mind and, understandably, Paula was quite shocked, although she agreed that the male cats were always troubling poor Queen—she was constantly being hounded by her own son, Inca, whose hormones were raging as he was coming into adolescence. In desperation, Paula asked if this situation could be turned around.

I told her that Queen may be better off where she is, and that if she did decide to return, she'd have to be desexed. Queen had made it clear to me that she wanted some girlie privileges, as she was constantly pushed out of sight by the males, including the new puppy. She didn't wish to be a new mother over and over again, but wanted instead to explore other avenues of life as a cat.

Paula rang me several weeks later to say that she'd seen Queen down the street, out the front of a house. She contacted the people that lived there and was pleasantly surprised to find they were a lovely couple that adored Queen and her four new kittens. Paula decided to honour Queen's decision and leave well enough alone. It was a hard thing to do, and I admire Paula for her generosity in putting Queen first.

41

Finally Free

BIRDS HAVE WINGS AND LOVE TO FLY, SO IF AN OPPORTUNITY TO escape presents itself, they'll take it. Even though they may have been indoors most of their lives, either in a cage or within the confines of certain rooms of a house, most birds long for freedom instinctively.

Mickey, a blue Budgerigar, spent the majority of each day in a small cage in the back of a hardware store, and was taken home each night after closing and brought back in the morning. This had gone on for four years. The owners of the shop, Rick and Helen, didn't want to leave Mickey at home as they thought he may be lonely. They were very kind, and they made sure Mickey had a chance to stretch his wings and fly around the back room at work a couple of times a week. They presumed Mickey was one happy Budgerigar.

Then one day Rick and Helen rang me in a terrible state. While Mickey was having his little fly around, a customer arrived and Rick went out front to serve him but didn't properly close the connecting door. Mickey managed to slip into the shop and from there he flew out the front door. Rick felt terribly guilty for his carelessness, and he and Helen desperately wanted to know if he was okay, as they feared for his safety.

When communicating with Mickey, straightaway I picked up on how resilient he was. I saw that he had managed to find food and water and was doing quite well, so that was the *good* news . . . but there was *bad* news. He had travelled far away and had no intention of returning, because he loved his new found freedom and being able to fly at will.

I obviously had to relay his words back to Rick and Helen, who were quite taken aback. They hadn't understood that his constant squawking was in protest at his living conditions. So it was farewell Mickey, and a lesson learnt by Helen and Rick.

Another case I remember well is George, an elderly gentleman with a Cockatiel named Rosie. George's wife had died five years previously and Rosie had been his sole companion for the past three years. She was both gentle and very attentive to George. Rosie happily travelled around the house on George's shoulder, rarely spending time in the elaborate cage he had bought for her. She'd stand on the dining-room table eating her food while George had dinner, with the pair of them chatting away.

George had three grown-up children and seven grandchildren and was quite often asked to babysit, as the youngsters loved spending time with him. One Sunday afternoon George was looking after the nine-year-old twin boys while their parents were househunting. The boys were happily out the back playing on their bikes when suddenly

George heard one of them scream. He immediately ran outside to see what the drama was all about.

George could see that one of the boys had fallen off his bike and was on the ground crying. As he ran over to assist his grandson, he suddenly realised that Rosie was still on his shoulder, and with that she took flight, no doubt upset at all the panic.

George first established that his grandson was okay and only shaken by the fall, but then kept watching out for Rosie. In horror he could see his bird heading for nearby trees. He ran towards the trees but by the time he got there Rosie was nowhere to be seen. To make matters worse, a storm which had been brewing all afternoon finally arrived with a vengeance.

Thunder, lightening and heavy rain were never a good mix for super-sensitive Rosie, and George knew this combo would only add to her already agitated state. He hurried the boys inside, then waited on the patio for Rosie. After calling her for more than an hour, with the weather deteriorating further, he feared the worst.

When his daughter and son-in-law returned home to collect the boys, they saw the sadness on George's face. They immediately went outside with him to try and find her. With no luck, they deeply felt his pain. The three of them put out flyers and posters, still hoping against hope that some good person may have found her.

George's daughter, Rhiannon, contacted me after being referred by a friend. George and I began a session, mindful that several days had past and there was no way of knowing how many kilometres Rosie could have flown. I connected with Rosie without any difficulty, but her energy felt very light and distant, which for me usually meant they had passed over, or were in a physically weakened state. It wasn't looking good.

I got right to it, asking Rosie what had happened that stormy night, and where was she right now. She explained she had been frightened when George rushed outside, and then took flight. She had never flown that far before and headed for the trees. Already quite disorientated, the storm frightened her even more and so she flew to the safety of denser trees. Unfortunately there were other birds sheltering there too, and they flew at her in a menacing way to convey that this was their territory. With that, she was chased for quite a distance, and a couple of her pursuers pecked at her wings, causing injury. When poor Rosie finally managed to escape, she was far away from home and had an open wound. As she told me this sad story, I recalled what it was like to be lost as a child. It's the worst feeling in the world.

Rosie had no idea how to get back to George, and was even more concerned about her damaged wing. It was very difficult to fly, so she had no choice but to stay put for a couple of days. Unfortunately in that time her wing worsened and she became ill with infection. Terrified and sick, she fell to the ground and died.

As her body was never found, George could never have known what had happened to her without my intervention, and he would have always wondered what had become of his beautiful Rosie. Even though his grief at the loss was almost unbearable, at least now he knew to stop looking for her. These days the buzz word is 'closure', and there's something to be said for it.

As I tried to comfort George, it was clear his sense of guilt over her being outdoors would perhaps take time to fade. From Rosie's perspective, there was no blame to be laid—it was just bad luck, along with rotten timing. It was nobody's fault.

There are many animals that have unfortunately passed over while being lost, and I've communicated with plenty of them. Some have succumbed to natural causes, others to physical injury. And even though it can be emotionally disturbing for their human families to learn this awful news, I know that it usually helps console people to know the truth, as painful as it is.

42

Wild Inside

CERTAIN MALE CATS SEE THEMSELVES AS HUNTERS AND adventurers, roaming great distances to fulfill this primitive need. What's fascinating is that they tend to widen their territory over time as they seek to discover what's out there in the vicinity. I liken these felines to cats in the wild, such as lions, leopards or tigers.

There are also those animals that choose to roam in order to select a mate for themselves. Again, certain aspects of their living arrangements are too limiting to enable this to happen naturally. People have asked me if it would make a difference if *they* were to procure a mate for their animal. It's an interesting question, and here's my response: although this works for many animals, for others it has to be the animal's choice; that's paramount to them.

This was the case for Rino, a male, caramel Burmese who left home one morning and wasn't seen for days. When Tina and her partner, Mike, reached me they were distraught with worry. I connected with Rino and discovered he'd taken off because he wanted to see what was out there in the wide world. He was also looking for a female to share his adventures.

When discussing this with Tina, she suggested they get a female Burmese, if this would solve the problem of Rino going walkabout. I took this idea to Rino, but he made it clear in no uncertain terms that he wanted to choose his own partner. He was a very confident, self-assured male who was on the prowl to select a suitable mate. So that was that. Rino did say, however, that if he went on a long enough adventure and still couldn't find a mate, he'd consider returning home, as he did indeed love Tina and Mike.

This of course was not what Tina wanted to hear, but Rino wasn't really offering a choice. He had shown me that he wasn't far away. As I explained to Tina, if you find him and bring him back, he'll just find a way to leave again until this quest is out of his system.

Rino had always been one very independent, confident cat. He had lived his life predominantly as an outdoor cat, but was locked in after dark, which is a responsible thing for cat owners to do. This was very distressing for Rino, as nights were when he wanted to establish his territory and go on the prowl. As difficult as this was, Tina agreed to be patient and see if he was going to return. I admired the good grace she showed in accepting the way things were.

There are times when we must accept that if animals don't return, then it may be that their desire to move on is for their own benefit. They have their own passions and desires and, just like us, they have a right to live their lives as they choose. Many have simply finished their teachings with us, and they are required elsewhere to assist others, or simply need to structure a new journey for their own enlightenment. For anyone who loves animals, this is a big lesson.

43

Happy Endings

LIKE EVERYONE ELSE, I'M A SUCKER FOR A HAPPY ENDING, AND that's why I want to share this story with you. A handsome brown rabbit decided to go walkabout—or should I say 'hop about'—one afternoon. His name was Cinnamon and he adored playing with his family, Roger and his two children, Benjamin and Lucy. He was a cheeky little fellow and they knew very well how much he loved to explore.

One afternoon they put him out in the backyard, as they routinely did, but on this occasion, when they went to bring him inside, he was nowhere to be found. Mysteriously, they couldn't find a hole or any other means by which he could have escaped. They thought the worst—he must have been stolen.

Roger contacted me as his children were distraught, unable to imagine life without their darling, floppy-eared friend. He'd been part of the family for a year.

It had been a week since he disappeared by the time I came into the picture, so I had no idea what I'd find out. I connected with Cinnamon, and what a character he was! He told me he'd simply decided to go on a bunny adventure, and with his determined nature, that is what he did.

He went beneath some shrubs along the back fence and dug his way into the neighbour's backyard. As he dug furiously, it filled up the hole on *his* side of the fence, which is why the hole was difficult to detect. Once in the next yard, he hid under some plants for a day or so as there were two small dogs who lived there. Cinnamon waited until they had gone inside before making a hasty escape.

He ran under the mesh gate at the side and sat under a leafy plant in the front yard to rest. It wasn't quite the adventure he had planned as there were cars and people everywhere. He wasn't sure which way to go, but didn't really want to confront those dogs while trying to get back home. So he made himself comfortable while planning his next move.

Before long a schoolboy walking past noticed him and slowly approached. Cinnamon wanted to make a run for it but when the boy pulled some food out of his backpack he couldn't resist. Cinnamon wasn't afraid, as children had always been kind to him in the past. He sat there nibbling his way through the food he'd been offered. The boy then picked him up and decided to take him home.

At this point I could sense they were travelling in a south–south-west direction. They seemed to go for a kilometre or so before reaching a house. Cinnamon showed me the boy putting him in the backyard with other rabbits who welcomed him into their playful group. Although he was having fun, he soon longed to be back home playing with Benjamin and Lucy.

I relayed this information to Roger, who had been frantically putting flyers around the place but, as it happened, not in the area described in my communication with Cinnamon. So he went out and did this immediately. In less than twenty-four hours, Roger phoned to say he'd located the runaway Cinnamon, safe and well in the company of six other rabbits. The schoolboy's mother had rung, apologising. She said her son was always bringing stray rabbits home, and that he'd meant no harm.

Of course Benjamin and Lucy were overjoyed to see Cinnamon, just as he was to see them.

One of my first lost animal cases was for my friend Gina who had a love bird. Gina phoned me frantically one day as her beloved Charlie had flown the coop. He was her pride and joy and they had a remarkably close relationship, so this was truly devastating for her.

Just to give you an inkling of the bond between them: Charlie was allowed to fly through the house at will, joining in any activities with Gina and he would sit on Gina's pillow at night while she read in bed. Charlie even loved sitting on Gina's finger while he untiringly groomed each and every one of her eyelashes! You could say they were very attached to each other.

One of their daily routines was his flight around the backyard, with Charlie flying from Gina's finger over to a bush or tree and then back. The routine was always the same and he never attempted to fly away . . . until one fateful day when things went horribly wrong.

On this occasion, a large black bird intercepted his short journey while he was flying back to Gina's finger. Charlie was so completely startled that he felt he had no other choice but to flee for his life. It all happened so quickly that Gina didn't even see in which direction he flew. He was just gone.

She desperately called and called him, as she ran from tree to tree, but there was no sign of him.

Charlie described the whole terrifying event to me and I really picked up on his fear. He showed me how he flew down the street and around a corner to escape the black Crow. He then revealed to me the woman he was with, letting me know he was safe and being cared for.

I relayed this information to a tortured Gina, adding that the house he was in was very close by. She flew into action (excuse the pun), putting flyers in letterboxes in the immediate area. Within a day she had Charlie back home, safe and sound.

The lady who had been looking after Charlie had seen one of the flyers and immediately phoned Gina. She had found him drinking from her dripping air conditioner. She noticed how tame he was, so she'd approached him. Charlie apparently jumped onto her finger and she was able to take him inside. She knew from his ease with people that he wasn't a wild bird. She felt sure someone must have been looking for him and had kept an eye out for 'lost' notices.

Reuniting people with their beloved animal friends in whatever way possible is a wonderfully rewarding experience. It's one of the joys of the work I do.

44

Captive or Free

HUMANS WERE ONCE WILD AND FREE. IN EARLY TIMES THEY roamed the earth, interacting effortlessly with other species. There existed an innate respect for the planet across the species, as it fed, sheltered, and provided them with life. Animals had close associations with humans, and were only slain for survival purposes. How wonderfully harmonious (and sensible!) this equilibrium between the humans, animals and the earth must have been.

The restrictions we've created through the centuries now affect all living creatures. These may be in the form of governments, religions, parents or employers, or the many accepted rituals in place in our society. Often we suffer self-imposed restrictions in our lives thanks to our limited thinking. We simply do not release ourselves to do the things we were destined to do. We should be more aware of our inner desires and those of others—including different species who may now depend on us. It takes all species for the planet to function and continue evolving.

Domestic or captive animals get few choices over the direction of their lives. Many are asked to spend their days in unnatural situations, such as living completely indoors or in a cage. When birds are in a cage they can't even do what all birds do, which is fly. That would be like binding *our* legs so we couldn't even walk, condemning us to a boring, stationery existence with nothing to do.

Think about horses boxed into small paddocks or stables where movement is limited, fully inhibiting their noble, athletic natures. I view horses as instinctually wild, rather than domesticated animals, and I have communicated with many horses that wish to be free to roam. People who have been very involved with horses know that there is a powerful sense of freedom in their nature, and it's sheer cruelty on our part to disregard that. Those horses that are reasonably happy to be in a domestic setting have revealed to me that fewer restrictions would improve the quality of their lives no end.

It's only right that the animals in our care are content. It's our responsibility. If dogs and cats are treated correctly they can truly have wonderful lives, and can attain something of the freedom and expression their species yearn for.

There are exotic animals, like pythons and lizards, who are often kept in small wooden or glass display cases for human enjoyment, with only artificial light for warmth and illumination. Movement is almost out of the question for some of these creatures, and very limited for others, depending on the size of the enclosure. A snake in the wild doesn't just curl up and stay in one spot for its entire life. With countless exotic animals kept in this way, the question for me is, is it right for them to be classified domestic in the first place? Why can we not be satisfied with the species that are content to live in domesticity and share our lives? Many of these animals' instincts, both genetically and anatomically speaking, will never be fulfilled or maintained in a captive environment. It can lead to inner torment.

Communicating with pythons such as Romy and Benson has given me great insight into their species. Romy, a large Diamond Python, and Benson, a Children's Python, were living with Sandy in an enclosure in her house. As it turned out, Sandy had quite a few questions for them both to make sure they were enjoying a healthy, happy life, so she contacted me. She particularly wanted to know how they felt about breeding, and whether she should provide them with suitable mating partners.

Romy was definitely the more dominant of the two, perhaps due to her size. She was confident and didn't hold back in conveying what she wanted. Benson on the other hand was more passive and easygoing. Their initial comments to me were to do with their displeasure at the endless barriers they encountered when moving around the small enclosure. They informed me that it should be more like their natural habitat. It was too bare, and didn't provide any privacy. The unfamiliar human noises and vibrations in Sandy's house also made them anxious, as they couldn't move away from them.

Romy and Benson felt humans make selfish decisions, with scant regard for other species. The pythons spoke too of suffering boredom due to lack of natural stimuli. Romy referred to the issues of natural light, seasonal changes and temperature, as these were the triggers for many of their physiological functions. The artificial light and heating were sometimes too constant in their enclosure, with the heat itself often too high for their comfort.

Their natural eating habits in the wild—finding and capturing prey—were far more stimulating than being given a dead animal in the enclosure, and they made that clear to me. They were missing the thrill of the chase and the opportunity to strategise.

I then conveyed Sandy's questions regarding mating and they replied that they wished to choose their own mate because, as they put it, mating is an instinctual occurrence and can't (or shouldn't) be decided by another. They also felt that the conditions in their enclosure did not offer the correct elements for happy mating.

I moved on from that to tell them that Sandy wanted to know why they didn't appear to appreciate being held. Benson spoke up, explaining that humans didn't seem to understand the musculature of snakes, which relies on surface area and tension. Apparently when Sandy picked them up with two hands in two different parts of their bodies and suspended them, they felt disabled and sluggish. It wasn't a pleasant experience, so sometimes they'd retaliate by snapping.

Snakes weren't really designed for human handling. Romy in particular didn't know why people had this great yearning to hold snakes in the first place. She knew Sandy felt tentative when handling her, which made two of them who were nervous! Romy told me she could get used to being handled if Sandy did it correctly, but not for long periods.

I appreciated Romy's frankness in making it clear that her genetic affinity with the wild would sometimes take over, which she expressed as resentment at being dominated by a human. Benson explained that, as snakes have a wild instinct, it would be helpful if this could be communicated to the human species, so they could better understand the way of snakes. He wanted me to get this message across to Sandy in particular, as he knew she was fascinated by them. Interestingly, Benson felt the reason for this was that Sandy has a deep, inner link with the wild, and is drawn to the idea of being free. She admires the snakes' sense of independence, just as she keenly values her own.

He went on to tell me he knows Sandy finds snakes beautiful as a species, and that he in his own way finds her beautiful. It got even more wondrous, for Benson explained that he regularly sent her pictures and feelings telepathically, but he knew that Sandy imagined these to be her own thoughts.

When I relayed this to Sandy she was excited by the fact that Benson was trying to communicate with her. I explained to Sandy that she needed to work on the stilling of her mind to create a mood of calmness. She tended to be a livewire and was rarely quiet, so this would be a challenge for her, but it was clear she couldn't wait to experience the world of animal communication and was keen to give it her best shot.

Our fascination with these wild animals surely can be fulfilled by viewing them in their natural environments. If we put them in cages, the initial fascination wears off and then the plight of these animals worsen. Many reptiles in particular are from geographic locations far from where they are housed, and if they should escape or be set free by people no longer wanting them, it could be disastrous—especially when you consider that some pythons grow several metres long.

There was a three-metre-long python found in the basement of a building in New York, and the fireman who came across this snake knew it had been in captivity as it seemed very familiar with humans. The type of python was not native to the area, so it had either escaped or been let go. The poor animal was unlikely to have found food in the basement, so it would have starved to death. And just think, if a python this large had come across someone's dog or cat, or even a small child, it could have ended in catastrophic circumstances.

If these animals were to breed in an area that was otherwise free of their species, think of the effect on the ecosystem. Competing with other animals for food, animals that were normally predators could now be prey. This is the type of problem that could wipe out whole species, which has already occurred in many countries around the world when non-indigenous animals have been introduced.

Before businesses consider selling animals as a money stream they must consider the environmental effects and ethics of doing so. One of my clients contacted me to speak with his lizards. David was faced with a problem that he hadn't anticipated. He had purchased two young Bearded Dragon lizards—a male called Grigor and a female called Lorika. They were brother and sister. He had had them for several months and all was going well, until the two weeks before his call.

David noticed on a couple of occasions that when he got home from work Grigor was uncharacteristically on the opposite side of the cage behind a rock. When he went to investigate he noticed blood in the enclosure. As David removed Grigor from the cage he saw that his tail was badly damaged. He wasn't sure exactly what had happened but immediately separated him from Lorika. He waited a few days and then placed Grigor back in with Lorika. After only a few hours he found Grigor in a similar condition.

David realised he would have to separate these two lizards indefinitely until he could find out what was going on.

As I communicated with both Grigor and Lorika, the story unfolded. They were both developing into sexual maturity. Grigor was making advances toward Lorika, which she did not welcome. The instinct to mate for Grigor was quite overwhelming, and Lorika was the only available female. Lorika recognised that he was her sibling, so she wasn't agreeable to mating with Grigor at all. Instinctually this did not feel right to her. The only way she could discourage his closeness was to lash out.

Lorika told me she was happy to breed, but not with him, and she was keen to know if more males of her species would become available. I told her I would need to check with David.

David couldn't believe what I was saying. He said he never would have picked that that was the problem. He knew then and there it was impossible to place them together again. They would need, at the very least, a mesh barrier between them.

As for mating partners David felt this would be difficult. If he arranged a male for Lorika, he may not be to her liking and then what would happen to the male? He couldn't keep all of the males. The same was true of females for Grigor. He decided to contact a reptile club to see if anyone else was looking for mating partners for their lizards. This way he could provide them both with partners and give them back to their people afterwards.

As you can see, even with the greatest intentions, living environments are sometimes highly unsuitable. It's very difficult trying to create a natural environment in an unnatural setting.

One of my early consultations with wild animals was for a woman named Roxy from Zimbabwe. She had rescued a lion cub, when he only three days old, from war veterans. This was a case of humans invading the animal's world. This poor creature would have died if Roxy hadn't stepped in and welcomed him to her plantation. Bones was now nine months of age and Roxy felt some sadness from him. She needed to know why, and to see if she could help in any way.

I connected with Bones and he came across as very strong and confident. He wanted to be heard. Bones said he knew who he was, and was very proud of it. He was a leader but didn't want to be the main lion in a pride. He mourned the loss of his family (his mother and siblings had died) and felt alone in a sense. He wished for a brother to walk with, side by side. The inner emotional scars of his turbulent start were still causing him pain. He asked why this devastating event had happened to him. I explained to him that humans sometimes get caught up in their own struggles and feel the need to fight.

Bones knew he was not like the other two lions, Savannah and Mambo, that lived on the plantation. He was an outsider and would never be like them. They had formed a bond with each other, and were quite happy to live in an enclosure. Bones relied more on Roxy for companionship, as she loved and accepted him. Bones was still unsure if his place was at the plantation at all. Maybe he wouldn't stay long, but right now it was where he was. He just knew he had survived for some particular reason.

The thought of venturing out into the wild held great fears for him, but he believed that one day he would want his own pride and family. The truth was, on the plantation he would always be alone. He felt lost and unsure of his direction, but he knew his instincts, when fully developed, would lead him to roam as a lion was meant to. Bones asked that when that time came, he be freed and released into a place safer than from where he had come.

Roxy said the responses from Bones had been one of the most incredible things that she had ever had the good fortune to experience. Everything she had suspected had been put into words. She pointed out that finding such a place for him would be extremely difficult. Natural landscapes are so scarce for the inner freedom these animals seek.

We have to respect and honour an animal's right to have independence and live their own lives where possible. Perhaps certain species need to be viewed and studied in the wild. Caging a human against their will is classed as imprisonment and has serious consequences. The same should apply for animals. If they don't have access to fresh air, exercise, a whole-food diet, natural exploration and of course independence, they flounder. If they are divorced from what is natural for too long, they may suffer from the same 'dis-eases' that people endure.

Perhaps *our* disconnection from nature needs to be viewed far more seriously so these issues can be resolved.

45

What Animals Tell Us

AS I'VE DESCRIBED, THERE IS MUCH TO DISCOVER FROM COMMUNING with animals who are no longer on earth—but I must emphasise that we can learn from them while they're still with us in the physical sense. Especially the wild animals. I can't overstate this: animals know what humans have forgotten, which is the importance of staying connected to your core or intuitive self. That means to remain grounded and in communion with all life.

Animals are masters of intuition. They have never been told that intuition doesn't exist, or that it's made up. Lucky them! Animals don't have any cultural limitations as people do; they communicate intuitively all the time within, and outside, their own species. Just think about the wonder and the majesty of that.

As far as I'm concerned, this could explain the odd ways animals can react to a new person, animal or situation they don't feel comfortable with. How many times have *you* been mystified with just such a scenario? Animals have also been known to alert their owner to an impending medical emergency, such as an epileptic fit. They can also predict natural disasters by changes in their behaviour before earthquakes, storms and volcanoes. This was indeed the case before the devastating 2004 tsunami. Animals were seen to leave the area and head for higher ground hours before it struck, and animals in zoos in the area wouldn't come out of their enclosures. Very few animals lost their lives in that tragedy, compared to the hundreds of thousands of people who were unaware of the imminent disaster.

The truth is that animals are in tune with the natural biorhythms of this planet, while we have lost the connection. In a changing world of technology—especially in western societies—people have also become more obsessed with their careers and material trappings, so being biorhythmically attuned goes by the wayside. By and large, we no longer know how to be still, and how to quieten our minds. A state of just *being* seems to be impossible for most people, but it's a necessity if you want to hear the inner you, and to find your connection to the natural world.

Minds are in a constant state of chatter with the incessant stimulation of computers, TVs, radios, iPods and all the rest of it, so the opportunity for peace is greatly reduced. People don't ever seem to be in silence, alone with themselves. This gives rise to increased stress and anxiety in our everyday lives.

Having high or unreasonable expectations of ourselves is another main cause of stress, but animals can show us to take what comes and work with it. They still manage to purr, wag their tails and make the most of any situation. Now that's certainly something to contemplate.

These days everyone is in a hurry. Particularly the younger set which prefers technological stimulants rather than a walk in the forest, being absorbed in a personal development book or just sitting by the ocean and watching an exquisite sunset. Perhaps they have had little opportunity to experience these things, to know the difference. Animals will always choose to be in natural, peaceful surroundings over settings that are noisy and congested.

Most people don't realise why they are not at ease with themselves or their environment. Or why they're constantly searching for something, anything, to make them truly happy. My belief is that, without knowing it, we're actually trying to find that lost connection. The connection that not only enables us to look inside ourselves, but to connect with everything in the universe for wholeness.

Here's an irony: more and more people look for solitude and serenity only in a place of nature. They'll spend thousands of dollars retreating to a tropical island or sailing down a picturesque fjord to try and maintain their sanity. Yet most of the human race are hell-bent on creating more cities and stimulants! Have we not yet worked it out? Happiness and serenity come from within; from what we create for ourselves. Being in these calm environments allows us to truly find and hear ourselves. Watch the animals in these natural environments and you will see inner tranquility in its purist form.

Animals can clearly show us what harmony is all about, and if you observe them closely, they sure seem to have everything worked out. Numerous species can live in one area and coexist without drama. They don't have wars—they spar merely to protect territories, and only to the death when it's necessary for survival. Once the sparring is over, a grudge or resentment isn't held; they simply walk away. Human wars, on the other hand, can go on for years, and hatred between people can linger long afterwards with long-term repercussions.

PART VIII

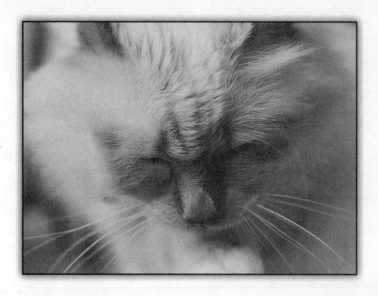

Love, Loss and Living in the Moment

46

Loved No Matter What

ANIMALS ARE ABLE TO SEE WHO WE TRULY ARE UNDERNEATH ALL the man-made trappings and, no matter what, they'll love and cherish us. They have an uncanny way of appealing to a side of us we often don't pay enough attention to. I'm talking about the part of us that wants to run free and have fun.

Animals don't worry about tomorrow; they're more preoccupied with right now. Because they share a very personal and spiritual relationship with you, they can teach you many oh-so-important lessons about living in the moment. I can assure you that if we didn't have animals in our lives, many of us would never delve deep enough to discover who we really are. We'd only be scratching the surface to our true existence.

Those people who are aware of this great truth know to trust and honour an animal's impeccable values. They may well open their hearts more fully to an animal, than to a human, because it feels so safe. An animal will love us no matter what, and expect very little from us. Even if they're mistreated at times, they'll still forgive and love you. Heavens, if we could practice this unconditional behaviour in our own lives, and convey this to others, imagine what could be achieved? This is totally unselfish, and that is something that is fading fast in our society.

I love the way animals can transform us back to innocence and into the child we once were, untouched by all the negative influences we've encountered through the years. As children, all our dreams seem possible, and everything is ahead of us; we are fearless. Sadly, we lose that along the way. For animals, this is their life-long philosophy. They are in a permanent state of optimism, always remaining in the present. Being able to look through the eyes of a child is what we are missing as adults, and it's a very big loss.

You know, we tend to fall into a rut very easily and just bumble along, imagining there will be time later to get around to what we truly want to do. It's funny (if that's the right word to use here) but 'later' never seems to come. If we are acting now on our experiences just think of the time we are saving longing for dreams to fall into place.

I remember speaking a few years ago with a man called John who was travelling the world, giving lectures on how to live your best possible life. He told me that for his research he had interviewed elderly people, and he was amazed that most of them didn't speak so much about what they'd accomplished, but rather about the things they had never managed to experience. There were many things they still felt they wanted to do, but due to failing health and waning vitality, time had beaten them. And they all just wished they'd thrown fate to the wind and had gone and done those things when they had the chance. Now, unfortunately, they lived in regret.

Animals don't experience this sadness because, as I said, they live in the moment and make the most of every opportunity available to them as it presents itself. Being so passionate about my work as an animal communicator certainly keeps me very busy. Consultations, healing animals, conducting workshops and writing books, to name but a few of my passions. There was a period when my husband was having to drag me away from my work, just to force me to make space for relaxation. This was around the time we adopted our first canine family member, Akeira.

I should say here that although a bundle of puppy joy, Akeira was quite a handful. My husband travels with his work, so whenever he went away, for Akeira it was just me. This meant playtime! I seemed to be constantly chasing her around the backyard, with my laundry pegs or my underwear firmly in her mouth! Initially it was an annoying distraction to my work, having a hyperactive puppy. On a couple of occasions I fell over chasing her. Akeira would just stop and look at me, as if she was laughing. She'd go through this funny routine, as if surrendering. Then, just when I was almost back on my feet, she was off again on another round of 'catch me if you can'. As I began to laugh, she'd run over to me and we'd rolled around on the grass together, tears rolling down my face.

It was during one of those moments, I realised this was exactly what I needed. It was like a huge release of bottled-up emotion. I had become so serious, and it was wonderful being silly for a change and having fun again!

Animals know we have failings, and they are there to help and guide us. I'm sure you've noticed that when you're upset, one of your animals will always come around to comfort you. They're able to sense our every emotion and will often see and know more about us than we do. As I've already indicated, there are times when our animal companions are reacting uncharacteristically because they're mirroring our illness or our behavior, in the hope we'll twig to what we're doing wrong. You learn so much about yourself during this process, although most often you won't even notice, thereby missing this incredible gift that's there for the taking.

Animals also teach us that life is a cycle, and death merely a transition to a rebirth or new life. They know that—they don't see death as the end. They understand at a deep level that they'll continue on afterwards. They just get on with the life they have now and make the most of every opportunity it has to offer. And if certain things don't work out, they're very unperturbed, moving on to the next event.

I've heard so many people say, 'In my next life I want to come back as a cat or a dog.' This is because they feel that these animals have such a relaxed and perfect existence. When animals are in a loving home, this is very true— eating, sleeping and having fun. If you think about it, life could be so much simpler now. Even though we have certain responsibilities, we tend to make things a lot more complicated than they need be. Perhaps if we didn't, more of us would be contented and grateful.

47

Losing an Animal

AS HUMANS, WE HAVE VARIOUS SPIRITUAL BELIEFS (OR NONE) ON the subject of death. Whatever we believe or don't, helps shape our reaction to death. There are cultures that celebrate death with a week-long party of singing and rejoicing, rather than with a formal funeral. They're celebrating that life, and giving the person a grand send-off into the spirit realms.

Some cultures believe in the afterlife. Those that don't will obviously have a totally different experience when death touches their lives. You also hear stories about people close to the end seeing a deceased relative in the room, as though someone is waiting to take them to the other side.

Near-death experiences are well documented, especially ones about being in a tunnel with a glowing light at the end. And when the person reaches the light, there have often been deceased relatives and friends to greet them. As they hadn't gone to the other side, but returned to the physical realms, we get to hear about what happened. Those who relate these stories insist they were told, 'Go back. It's not your time.'

My first experience with the death of an animal was with my childhood dog, Slasher, who I talked about earlier. The gorgeous, unforgettable Slasher, my steadfast buddy. We had a very close relationship and, naturally at fourteen years of age, I didn't have a great understanding about death and dying. My views and beliefs were inclined to come mostly from family and friends, and death seemed very final.

I must admit, though, throughout my childhood I'd go off by myself a great deal and talk to God, unicorns, flying horses and the like. It was my secret world. Deep down I knew there was so much I still had to discover, especially to do with matters of spirituality.

One day I came home from a day at the beach with my friends and as I walked into the kitchen my mum looked at me with sorrowful eyes. I knew instantly something was wrong, but didn't imagine it was about Slasher. Not my beautiful Slasher. As Mum told me he'd been hit by a car at the front of our house earlier that day, I let out a long, loud wail.

I ran into the backyard in disbelief looking for him. Even though I was spared the anguish of seeing the actual accident, I wasn't ready to see his body, covered by a tarpaulin, and didn't lift it. I simply fell to my knees and cried and cried, as I had just lost my closest friend.

Later that day the family held a service and backyard burial for Slasher to honour his presence in our lives. We acknowledged through our tears that at least he died doing what he loved best: roaming the streets, visiting the neighbours.

My next canine companion wasn't until I was in my early twenties. His name was Winston and he was a Maltese Terrier.

We were devoted to each other. When he was eight years old, I moved out of the family home to buy my own house, and as the property didn't have fencing, my mum suggested leaving Winston with her until my place was secure.

I visited him every day, and he'd be waiting patiently by the front door until my car pulled up. He had always made me feel so special, as I did him. Winston had constantly showed me what loyalty and commitment were all about, making him the perfect companion.

When he was ten years old he developed a heart condition that required daily medication. As I was once again working full-time, my mum suggested it would be better for him to stay with her, rather than live at my new property. Mum was home during the day and could give him his medication and keep an eye on him. Although wanting him with me, I knew these arrangements were best for him. I still visited him every day of course, and he stayed with me at the weekends, so I remained very much in his life.

One night while out with friends my family called me on the mobile phone to tell me that Winston was very ill. He was having difficulty breathing. I rushed over and we took Winston to our vet. He was examined immediately, and the prognosis was not good. The vet said his heart was failing and there was fluid on his lungs. And the worst news of all was that nothing could be done.

Winston was on oxygen but still struggling, and I couldn't bear to see him in such a state, knowing there was no hope. I was left with no alternative but to have him euthanised to end his suffering.

Through the tears and saying my goodbyes, the vet administered the injection while I held him. He gave one last whimper as his body went lifeless, and I had this incredible yearning to go with him.

I wasn't sure where he was going, but that didn't seem to matter, just as long as we were together. The thought of him wandering around, lost in the darkness, was weighing me down like a boulder. Somehow I knew deep inside me that he was on his way to a place of love, and that he'd be okay. It was a gut feeling.

I understand now why so many people contact me to communicate with their loved ones once they've passed to the other side. They want to know where they go and what they do there. They want to know if anyone had met them on the other side. Others might be curious as to whether animals have a soul. For me, it's wonderful to be able to convey the answers to these questions direct from their beloved animal companion on the other side.

What I've learnt in communicating with animals after they've crossed over is that they go to a place of joy, lightness and beautiful visions. They're often met by angels or by human family and animals they've known on earth who have already passed. They never travel there alone, but with loved ones or beings of light, and are extremely well cared for.

This knowledge has been the most wonderful comfort to me, and it should be to you too. We're often faced with losing our animals through old age or illness, and I want you to know that even during those final hours or days when there might be great pain and suffering, the animals are able to distance themselves from the present circumstances and to transport themselves into a different state of consciousness. Once there, they no longer feel pain to the same extent.

Once the physical body is no longer present, the soul essence is forever universally present. And this essence remains close to the earth plane for some time, while the soul is released and prepares for the transition. Once the transition is complete, they're always watching over their human loved ones.

It's a lovely image, isn't it? And one that gives me infinite reassurance. Many, many animals have described to me their journey to the other side. For instance, an enlightened Golden Retriever, Raj, told me that as his soul essence left his physical body, he walked light and free toward an arched bridge over a glistening stream. A pure white angel stood either side of the bridge, above them a stunning rainbow formed a semicircle over the bridge. On the other side was a meadow of soft grass surrounded by sweet-smelling pine trees and brightly coloured flowers.

As Raj crossed the bridge, an elderly lady walked toward him. It was Ethel, the much-loved grandmother of his human family. Beside her stood a brown Beagle, his companion in a previous life time! As Raj met them, the three of them crossed the bridge together into the spirit realms and he experienced the joy and freedom he knew had been waiting for him.

Animals have also described for me the actual process of transition into the realms. It entails a cleansing and purifying of their energy or soul body as they leave their physical body. The spirit realms are of a higher vibrational frequency than here on this earth, so changes to their energy systems are required. If they were very ill or had a karmic effect in this life, then the cleansing process may take longer. In any case, once free of the physical body and purified, their spirit is light and free once more.

Gemima, a petite Chihuahua, was extremely gentle, and utterly devoted to her person, Bill. Bill and Gloria had been married for years when they adopted Gemima from an animal shelter. She was two years old and full of energy, and she went on to live a long and happy life with Bill and Gloria, bringing much joy into the family. And they loved her right back.

Sadly, when Gemima was twelve years old she succumbed to an illness and had to be euthanised. Bill was not coping with the loss of his much-loved companion, as they had been inseparable for years. To be without her now was incredibly painful and he longed to know if she was okay, and where she had gone.

I discovered there was a karmic link between Gemima and Bill. In a past life they had been twin brothers, separated at twelve years of age, never to be reunited. They had always pined for each other and each wondered what had become of their other half. Eventually the twin who Bill had been in that past life learnt that his brother had died from the Plague, and he felt guilty he'd hadn't died too. It's called survivor's guilt, and he never rose above his sadness at not having been there to support his brother in his time of need.

Gemima had come back into Bill's life again to replace that love and support which had been lost, to teach him about dealing with loss and ultimately about being able to move forward. This time, Bill was present to support Gemima through her entire illness, and was there at the end for her.

From the afterlife, Gemima was so pleased to be able to convey this information to Bill, in the hope he'd now move on with his life. Thanks to Gemima, Bill was set free, understanding that death is a natural occurrence, and not meant to hold us back in our quest for knowledge and enlightenment. He was overwhelmed when I explained everything to him, because he previously had no way of knowing about the link between the two of them in the past.

Bill realised how important it was to honour Gemima's memory and sacrifice, and to act on the lesson. He decided there and then to make every effort to learn from this and move into the next phase of his journey. He's convinced, as am I, that he'll be able to prevent Gemima from suffering again in a future life, by embracing what she has taught him.

Gemima also allowed me to revisit the intense cleansing and purifying she went through in order to remove the heavy karmic influence and her severe illness. Shedding this physical body had been quite a process for her. It had certainly taken longer than the purifying many other animals had described to me for Gemima to move into the light and beauty that was her right. She asked me to share this exquisite experience with Bill, to help him along the path of his growing development.

It's helpful to understand that animals don't experience the dying process as we do. As a dog once said to me, *Life is merely a transition, ready for the next exciting journey.* Animals know that their spirit never dies, but rather lives on through eternity.

What we humans miss most about our deceased animals is their physical presence. We miss being able to hold them and stroke them and interact with them in a physical sense. This is because we are a spirit in a physical body having a physical experience. It's comforting to know that, although their *physical* form is gone, the spirit and love of your animal friends are with you always. The bond of deep love and devotion will never be broken, as it surpasses time and space. The cherished memories are never forgotten.

I want you to understand something incredibly important here: there is only a veil between us and the spirit realms, so we can sense our animals, if we want to. It may not be in the same way we experienced them when they were alive. Nevertheless we can still communicate with them. We are so used to the physical touch of our animals, that it's difficult to be satisfied with this more subtle, yet every bit as real, intuitive sensing. But all you need is an open heart and mind, and the link will be there.

All I'm saying is, it's possible! And the potential rewards are immense.

Many people glimpse their deceased animals fleetingly, out of the corner of their eye. Others may see an impression in the bed which was their favourite place to sleep. Dreams are another way to reunite with your loved animal, as it's in this state of sleep that the realms are easily reached. The same is true when we dream of our deceased human relatives. They convey messages; or often the dream we are visualising is actually happening in a different consciousness. Either way, be on alert and expect the unexpected.

48

They Know It's Time

BELIEVE IT OR NOT, ANIMALS ARE BORN KNOWING ABOUT THE afterlife. They understand they'll eventually be returning home, as I found out through King, a gallant white stallion.

His guardian, June, had been given King from a horse rescue centre. She was a woman with a big heart, who had already saved many horses from traumatic circumstances. Sadly though, she felt King's condition was far beyond a recovery. June came to me for help because she wanted to be sure she was making the right decision about euthanasia for this noble beast.

Like me, June holds the strong view that euthanasia is the ultimate act of love and kindness; that we're acting selflessly in giving what is best for another. King was extremely emaciated through neglect and was so tired. He knew at a very deep level his journey had come to an end, and he was actually looking forward to the freedom and joy that awaited. I was able to confirm with King that he was more than ready to leave this world.

When I gave this information to June, she then knew what she had to do: she called for the vet to assist him on his way. As King fell into his final sleep, June was amazed at how calm he was, as though he was effortlessly surrendering to his next journey into the realms. She said it was one of the most beautiful experiences she'd ever encountered.

When I contacted King shortly after his passing, he clearly conveyed that, as he left his body, he saw a waterfall of white light in front of him. As he walked through it, he grew the most magnificent white wings, took flight, and began to soar towards the heavens. He told me how wonderful it was to be light once again, and free of the burdens of illness and pain of the earth plane.

As King went beyond the clouds, he landed on a golden path, where his spirit horse mother was waiting for him, and they continued on together into the realms. And just think: it was June who took the action that allowed King to soar when he was ready to go. Without her generosity, his flight into the light would have been delayed.

When I was in my early twenties, the same day as I brought home my Maltese Terrier, Winston, I also got Misty, an incredibly beautiful Chinchilla. She was the smallest of her litter and I still remember seeing her sitting there on the couch, with a big pink ribbon around her neck. Although only eight weeks old, she sat there confident and amazingly relaxed. Very little phased this small bundle of white fur.

Misty was a completely indoor cat who loved the comforts of her new home and quickly settled in when I moved away from my family and out on my own. Above all else, Misty was elated at now having a house to herself, away from the hectic barking of the dog. She became my best friend and companion during those years we spent time alone together. I'd arrive home from work and, while I was changing out of my work clothes, she'd saunter into the bedroom and sit right in front of me. I'd ramble on about my day, and she'd casually tilt her head to one side, taking in all my chatter. Then as soon as I'd finished my conversation, she'd get up, walk off and wait for me in the kitchen.

My little mate was so calming to be with, and seldom demanding. The perfect companion. And on her rare visits to the vet, they were amazed that Misty would sit on my lap in the waiting room so composed, no matter how many other cats or dogs were around her. Even in the examination room she was unperturbed by whatever procedure she was having. Then, while I'd be settling the account, she'd perch happily on the reception desk, enjoying attention from all the staff. She was unlike any other cat I had ever come across.

As it happened, it wasn't until she was just over seventeen years of age that I was intuitively drawn to leave my home and venture to a city on the other side of the country. As I mentioned, I knew the move was right for me, but my concern was that it would be too great a change for Misty at her age. All things considered, I figured it would be best if I could find a suitable place for her, rather than cart her to a new life so far away. As she had lived at my mother's previously, I thought that may be an option, but unfortunately Mum had a new cat of her own, who didn't get on with Misty—so that was that.

It wasn't long before my options for her slowly dwindled. I therefore decided to postpone my yearning for this new destination until it was her time to leave this earth. I felt I could never abandon my best friend, nor would I want to be without her.

A few weeks later, I woke early one morning to get ready for work. Coming out into the living area I noticed blood spots on the carpet. I immediately looked under my foot and around my body, thinking I may have scratched myself. As I investigated the carpet more thoroughly I noticed that these spots led in a particular direction. I followed them and they took me from the bed in the spare room out into the living area, and finally into the laundry.

I started to panic, thinking there must be a problem with Misty. I called and called her, while hurriedly running around the house to find her. Eventually she strolled out looking her calm self. I picked her up, examining every part of her body for evidence of bleeding. There was nothing. I began to clean up all the blood spots and she followed me, seeming bewildered about all the fuss.

I decided to check her kitty litter—and sure enough there were blood spots. I immediately feared she was having kidney problems. I rushed her to the vet and they placed her on a drip and performed a blood test. When the results came back several hours later it was true: she was in renal failure.

The vet was puzzled, because to look at her, she was absolutely fine. Normally, with the levels that were showing in her blood, she should have appeared very ill. I left her at the vet overnight and when I picked her up in the morning she was once more the picture of health. The vet said: 'Look, as long as she's going along fine, there's nothing more we can do for her, other than have her permanently on a drip in case she should dehydrate.'

There was never evidence of blood again and things pretty much went back to normal. Then a few weeks on I saw Misty sitting beside the dining room table with her eyes all drawn and the pupils enlarged. I knew that look of dehydration, and it always frightens the heck out of me. I rushed her to the vet and was told a decision had to be made. I couldn't believe it. It all happened so fast.

I phoned my family so they could be with me at this heart-wrenching time, and with them to support me I held Misty in my arms as she went peacefully to sleep and on to heaven. It was a devastating time and grief was upon me for many months.

I eventually followed my intuitive path, sold my house, and relocated, suspecting that Misty chose to die to allow me to continue my journey. She knew I wouldn't leave until she had gone to the realms—so that is what she did. Our beloved animals will never allow themselves to hold up your eternal journey.

What a selfless sacrifice Misty had made for me. I would like to honour her in this passage for her noble sacrifice, which will never be forgotten.

49

Your Animals Live On

ANYONE WHO HAS EVER LOVED AN ANIMAL WILL BE DEEPLY affected by their loss, no matter what the circumstance. When Tamara contacted me, her brown Staffi, Rufus, was fast deteriorating with cancer. She needed to know if his time had come, as she didn't want him suffering unnecessarily.

I appreciated that it was very difficult for Tamara to even ask this question, as he was her soul mate. Tamara was a brilliant counsellor, specialising in grief, but couldn't seem to help herself in the same way. The situation with Rufus was too close—meaning that emotion was clouding her ability to make decisions. Her heart was in pain, and as well as coping with her own ordeal, she was trying to assist Rufus with his.

Rufus told me he knew he had to go, but didn't wish to leave Tamara. He wanted me to tell her he'd remain close to the physical plane, to help her with the grieving process. Once again I was learning that death does not, and cannot, completely sever a great bond based on mutual love. Rufus also wanted Tamara to know he had enjoyed helping create a stabilising energy in their home, conducive to her healing and counselling work.

Patients had shattered lives when first coming to Tamara, but after receiving her various treatments, they left feeling more balanced and able to cope with the world. Her gift was great indeed.

As I delved deeper in my communication with Rufus, I discovered they had made a contract before either of them even came into this life, and now he wanted to remind her of this. This contract was to fulfill a planetary obligation, as well as one of personal enlightenment. And he made it clear to me that this entire adventure had been a pleasure for him from start to finish.

Life is meant to be fun, and experienced fully with each breath, Rufus said. He then asked that Tamara made sure she didn't allow her own light to dim while assisting others. Wow! What a powerful message to give to the one he loved.

Rufus wanted to continue assisting Tamara's patients from the spirit realms. So he requested that Tamara leave his dog bed in her consulting space, as she had always done. This would signify that his work with her would go on.

As Tamara fought back the tears, Rufus asked me to assure her that he wasn't afraid to walk 'home', knowing they'd work together again. He could see the channel of light forming for his departure, and knew he'd be welcomed by many when he got to the other side. He was looking forward to seeing old friends once more. With that, he bid farewell to his mum Tamara, and told her that he would love her forever. I'll never forget Rufus.

Suki, a darling Siamese, was reaching old age when we met. Aloof by nature, she was at times amazingly affectionate and attentive when it suited her. Typical of many felines, she ran the roost and had Kathryn, her owner, fitting in around her moods.

Several years earlier she'd had signs of skin cancer around her mouth and nose, but with treatment it all seemed to have cleared. When Kathryn contacted me, Suki was suddenly having bouts of bleeding from the nose, so it looked like the trouble had returned.

Kathryn wanted Suki's point of view as to the amount of treatment she wished to endure, which was such a loving thing to do. With intuitive scanning I saw right away that the cancer had returned. Suki made it clear to me that her body was giving up and she didn't have long before her return 'home'. She preferred to deal with the bleeding herself and didn't want Kathryn making a fuss around her. Even though there was often a burning sensation in her nose, Suki felt she could deal with this, and insisted she didn't want any further treatment. Rather, she preferred to let nature take its course.

Kathryn honoured Suki's wishes, although naturally it was difficult for her not to make a fuss. In the days that followed, Suki became much weakened from the cancer, until one day Kathryn came home to find Suki had passed away, curled up in a ball on her bed. She had obviously decided it was time to go. Kathryn, although grief stricken, felt blessed that my involvement had given her a chance to say goodbye, and she was comforted too in knowing what was on Suki's mind as regards to the end of her life.

Suki communicated with me after she had passed, insistent I let Kathryn know she had made it 'home' safely, and that she was free of her cancer now and in perfect form. I picked up too from this gorgeous creature that she remained mystified as to why humans fight so hard to stay on earth when the quality of life has clearly gone. Suki spoke to me with feeling about how dying is all part of the divine plan.

Kathryn asked me to tell Suki how much she loved her, which I did. But as Suki was now in the spirit world I knew that she could hear for herself the loving words Kathryn spoke.

Animals certainly provide us with great insight and a different understanding of the death and dying process. Listening to them at this deep level can help to alleviate the fear most of us have around this emotive subject.

50

How to Say Goodbye

EVEN THOUGH LIFE AND DEATH ARE ONE CONTINUOUS CYCLE, when our animals depart it can leave us with a lonely, empty feeling. My heart goes out to anyone who's been through such sadness, and my advice is this: when you're full of grief at the loss of your beloved animal friend, close your eyes and picture them clearly in your mind. Send them thoughts, and visualise messages of love. This will give you a clear connection, and you'll always know you can reach them.

Then open your eyes and look up at the sky to clouds or to the stars, and remind yourself that one day you'll be reunited with them. Farewell your beloved animals when they pass away and pay homage to their loyalty to, and love of you in life. I'm a great believer in giving them a fitting tribute. It's our way of showing how much we care, and that they'll never be forgotten.

Animals have described to me suitable ways of showing them our admiration at this sad time, such as burying them beneath their favourite tree or amongst brightly coloured flowers. Or you could place their precious ashes in an urn you can keep, so they will forever be with you, no matter how many times you move house.

I can assure you, animals have little concern for their physical bodies once they have passed over, as it's only a vessel to hold the soul. However, they'll take the opportunity when it arises to tell a communicator their ideas on ideal places for their bodies or ashes. Animals with their unique sensitivity understand that people need to have a place to openly express their love and their loss, and that this helps them attain a sense of closure. Holding a service can be incredibly healing (I know this from my own life) and it's a chance to reflect on special memories. A small prayer written from the depths of your heart to your beloved animal is another way to express your love. An example of this could be:

An Honouring Prayer

This is to honour my beloved [insert name of your animal].

Our love began the day you came, and continued to grow day by day,

You opened my heart, filling my life with happiness and joy,

Forever unconditional, and shining like a bright star in my life,

You have changed my world and you will be forever etched in my heart.

Love you now and always, until we meet again.

You could also erect a small shrine in a favoured spot in your home. Perhaps place a photograph next to their ashes if you are keeping them. You can maintain this shrine for as long as you like—and don't let anyone tell you 'You should be over the loss by now!' It's none of their business.

I can tell you, however, that animals don't like us to grieve, as this saddens them. Instead, they wish us to remember and celebrate all the joyous times they shared with us. You see, animals are extremely positive in the way they view death and dying.

51

Love at First Sight

WHEN ERIC AND ANDREA TOOK THEIR TWO CHILDREN TO THE animal refuge, they found love at first sight. After passing many dogs, they came upon Ruby: two twinkling, black eyes looking back at them, surrounded by her soft curly black Poodle hair. Instantly, they knew Ruby would be a part of their family. They scooped her up, excited about their new addition, but when they got Ruby home she was very quiet and rather anxious.

With their loving care and patience, however, Ruby soon proved to be the most energetic and playful member of the household. Ruby, along with Eric and Andrea's two children, would play for hours. She adored her new home and her family, so it was tragic when, after only five wonderful years of sharing their lives, Ruby was diagnosed with liver cancer. It was devastating for the family, who were left with only a few weeks with their dear pet before she deteriorated to such a point where there was no other choice but to euthanise.

The vet came to their house and Ruby was farewelled by her loved ones.

At this dreadful time for all of them, Andrea contacted me as she felt it was important to know where Ruby would like her ashes kept. She told me that the family was finding it very difficult without her. Ruby had always been a part of the most important events of the family's lives, and beautiful soul that Andrea was, she wanted to make sure that Ruby was involved in deciding where her ashes were to be laid to rest.

When I connected with Ruby, I understood what a sense of humour she had. She immediately began chatting away and I could feel the electricity of her energy. Ruby made me think that I should already know the answer to the question of where her ashes should be placed: *In the living area of course. I want to be right in the middle of everything—so that's the ideal spot.*

Andrea began setting up a small table against the living-room wall where everyone could see her photograph and her ashes. Each day she'd place a fresh rose there, and she reported back later that this had helped the family enormously.

When Bianca lost Milo, her German Shepherd of fourteen years, the grief was overwhelming. Milo had been ill for some time but this hadn't prepared Bianca for when he finally passed away. Milo had always been a carefree, playful dog, even into his senior years, and it was only in the final months he became quiet and listless, until finally passing silently one night whilst everyone was asleep. Bianca asked me to communicate with Milo to learn of his wishes, whether he wanted to be buried or cremated, and just where he'd prefer his final resting place to be.

Milo was clear: would I tell Bianca to bury him under the old almond tree in the backyard. He remembered Bianca always commenting on the beautiful pink flowers in spring, so it would be perfect. And he knew Bianca would need a physical location to visit for a time, thus allowing the healing to begin.

As many people are at a loss without the physical contact, a grave or shrine seems to help, just as it does when we're grappling with the loss of a much-loved person. It gives us a point of contact, although these honourings are more for *our* benefit than for our animals'. And they know that, but even in death and beyond animals consider how they can assist and give us love.

When animals are gravely ill and you know time is short, don't hesitate to express your love for them completely. Animals are amazingly intuitive, and they can hear your words and feel your heart.

Brigitte and Paul had been married three years when they had Bonnie join the family. Bonnie, a very energetic King Charles Spaniel, brought fun and laughter into the house, sharing in everything they did—holidays included. When Bonnie was struck down with pneumonia, Brigitte and Paul were frantic with worry. She wasn't responding to the medication and, at the vet's surgery, began to deteriorate rapidly.

The vet came to them with the bad news that it was unlikely she'd pull through, and this was when Brigitte and Paul came to me in the hope of conveying all their love and certain other thoughts to Bonnie.

Bonnie's message back to them was very clear. She reminded them how much fun they'd all had together.

That this illness had been such a short part of their shared existence, so they must not dwell on it; they should think instead about the amazing memories she'd take to the spirit realms with her. And that if she knew they were happy, this would help to ease her transition.

As hard as it was, Brigitte and Paul brought a stack of happy photographs into the veterinary surgery and talked to Bonnie about the great times they had, depicted by each photo. They swear they saw a hint of a smile and then, with her paw resting on Brigitte's hand, Bonnie was gone.

Don't wait until your wonderful companions are sick or deceased before you truly express how you feel. This is also true of the people in our lives. When was the last time you said, 'I love you' to someone you love? Or spoke of how appreciative you are that this person is a part of your life?

I sometimes think it's easier to say and show this to an animal than it is to other people in our lives. Usually because animals accept these gestures without question or suspicion. They won't ask us why, or ask us to tell them more, they will just lovingly take whatever we are offering with gratitude.

There's a lesson there!

We have our beloved animals for such a short time. Make every minute fulfilling and joyful. They are truly a blessing each and every day. If you have never shared your life with an animal then you have certainly missed out on some of the most amazing experiences of love and learning.

52

If Only

IT'S REASSURING TO KNOW THAT ALTHOUGH THEIR PHYSICAL form is gone, the spirit and love of your animal friends are with you always. The bond of love and devotion will never be broken.

Rob and Amanda received a wonderful little dog from the pound called Sprooker. He was a real trickster, being full of adventure and willing to try anything, and he made them laugh often. Not surprisingly they absolutely idolised him. They decided to take him on holidays with them when visiting friends, knowing Sprooker liked being in the car, and loved being anywhere they were.

The holiday was proving a great success, with Rob and Amanda's hosts falling for Sprooker's charms too. Typical Sprooker, he was champing at the bit to go off on his own exploring, but Rob and Amanda worried that as they were in a place foreign to him, he may lose his way.

One night they went out to dinner with their friends, leaving Sprooker tied up outside for the couple of hours they'd be away. He was under cover on the verandah, which Rob had checked thoroughly, making sure the area was safe. He even checked the rungs of the verandah surrounds to reassure himself that Sprooker couldn't slip through. All seemed fine, so they said goodbye to him and left for the evening.

Upon returning several hours later, Rob went to unleash Sprooker and was stunned in horror at the sight that greeted him. Sprooker had managed to squeeze through the narrow rungs and, because he was tied up, had hanged himself. Rob and Amanda were in extreme shock and distress, not only with having to deal with his death, but also with the guilt of making a decision that led to his demise.

Rob contacted me for a consultation to try to make some sense of what had happened. As soon as I connected with Sprooker I knew the words of this very special animal would soothe their souls.

Sprooker explained his realm was not for the foolhardy. It was for those who wished to step out and see further than the horizon. Sprooker said the adventure of life cannot be achieved within a comfort zone. Adventure is a journey of discovery. And how true that is.

Sprooker realised that Rob and Amanda were together for a distinct purpose, but life had begun to stagnate for them. He was the catalyst they needed for a renewed life. I sensed Sprooker was of fox energy and that he'd gone back to his dimensional world. Sprooker needed to show them the way, for that is the way of the fox. The fox outwits the humans in the hunt because humans tend not to look past their nose. They only see part of the picture, so foxes are always one step ahead, and they'll make you go that one step further, if you want to reap the reward. Sprooker was light again and on the job of his dimensional responsibilities. For the fox never rests.

Sprooker said that his transition to the spirit realms was very quick and easy. He felt catapulted into the heavens like a comet. He told me it was fun. But as he looked back toward his lifeless body, he knew the grief it would cause.

He directed his message to Amanda for a moment and said the beauty he saw in her eyes penetrated his very soul. He said it is time for both Amanda and Rob to keep the light shining and so create greater luminance together. A light was clearly seen by him between them.

Sprooker's incessant love for adventure unfortunately led to his end. He believed that even if death is imminent, it's always worth taking the risk. To be truly alive is to follow your heart and dreams. He said the dreams are within your heart, and to never allow an obstacle to prevent you from reaching that dream.

Sprooker wanted them both to know he had loved the years spent with them. He asked me to thank them for making life such fun, and for seeing the beauty within him. He directed me to tell them to honour his memory, and in return he promised to look in on both of them from time to time, just to make sure their path is always well lit, and its direction easily visible. His heart truly belonged to Rob and Amanda, and this would forever bind them together.

The message from Sprooker had a profound effect on Amanda and Rob, as I knew it would. They not only now saw Sprooker in a different light, but they also had clarity surrounding the reason of his death. They finally understood the depth of what Sprooker had taught them in such a short time. For Rob, this allowed his guilt to lift, and he was keen to learn from the wise words of Sprooker. Amanda, on the other hand, felt relieved he was happy and that he'd be by their side throughout life.

There are plenty of situations surrounding an animal's death that create sadness and guilt for their people. When an animal appears unwell, or decides not to eat, the decision to take them to the vet immediately, or wait a day or so to watch for improvement, can prove critical. And of course in many cases, there have been false alarms, so this may well result in a delay in getting to the vet the next time round. For others, such a delay is finance based—let's wait and see, and that way we may avoid unnecessary expense. There's no doubt it's sometimes difficult to know what to do when an animal is poorly. We can all be wise after the event, but that doesn't help.

Jessica had an extremely verbal cat called Yuri, who was a four-year-old chocolate point Siamese with a dominant attitude. He'd constantly walk around the house yowling and making demands. Bossy as all get out! Being the only cat, he had little competition and thrived on the verbal acknowledgement he got back from Jessica.

On this particular occasion his yowl was much louder and more frequent than usual, and Jessica was aware he'd barely eaten the entire day. Actually there was another time earlier when Yuri hadn't eaten for two days and he was completely fine—so she wasn't panicking. Jessica tended to ignore his yowling even though it was quite persistent, but by the second day his yowl became a scream and he still hadn't eaten, so Jessica became concerned and took him to the vet.

Upon examination, the vet told Jessica he had a blockage in the bowel and it could prove fatal. They would need to put him under anaesthetic to clear it.

Feeling really anxious, Jessica nonetheless went on home after the vet promised to ring her later with a report on how Yuri was doing. Unfortunately, when that call did come it was to tell her Yuri had passed away under the anaesthetic. It seemed that things were a lot worse than first anticipated, because the blockage hadn't been caught early enough. You can imagine the shock for Jessica. It had all happened so fast.

She spoke with me over the phone, desperate to be consoled over the guilt she felt. Jessica felt she should have taken Yuri to the vet sooner and also waited with him. The catastrophe was compounded by the fact that she didn't have the chance to say goodbye. She felt if she had acted differently, she could well have saved his life. I explained that she'd had no way of knowing, and that blaming herself for what could have been wouldn't help at all.

It's all a learning curve, and that's why we're here. This feeling of guilt happens to so many people when their animals pass away while at the vet's, especially during an operation. It makes it so much more difficult if you beat yourself up for not having stuck around during that crucial time. Of course, you would want to be with your best friend when they passed—it's only natural—but some things, unfortunately, are out of our control.

Animals have shared with me that they have *chosen* to pass when their person wasn't there. They felt it would be far less painful for the ones they love, rather than having them witness the event. They always have our welfare foremost on their minds.

53

A Lost Love

I HOPE IT'S BECOMING CLEAR WHY I'M ADDRESSING THE EMOTIVE topic of what happens when our beloved animals pass away. There's so much we humans can learn. By telling you what I now know, I hope you'll discover how to get through the sadness and the loss without staying stuck in grief forever. As I've indicated before, it's very difficult for us as our animals' guardians to make that final decision to have our friend put down, and yet we know deep down that because of illness or old age, their suffering should not continue.

The questions that constantly come up when people contact me over this issue are: Is this the right time to euthanise? Is it too soon? Will I ever get over the guilt of making this decision? Will my beloved animal hate or blame me for making this decision? Those who have asked have all made the tough call to euthanise based on love and compassion. Nothing else.

On the other hand, there are of course decisions that are sometimes made to euthanise unnecessarily—although I've never personally been involved in such a case, either before or after the event. I'm referring to people who, without reason or good intent, willingly have an innocent, healthy animal put to death just for the sake of convenience. To me this is horrendous, and those who do it need to look seriously at what this says about their character. And I'll tell you something even more chilling: these animals *know* the decisions have been made callously. Yes, they know.

In my experience, animals who are loved and share a special relationship with humans will never blame you for your decision when it's made from a place of love. They understand how difficult it is and that the decision came from the heart, and with the best of intentions. If this comes up in your life, you might want to consult a communicator if you would like the animal's viewpoint, which would then remove the onus from you entirely, giving all the power to the animal in question.

Riley was an event horse for most of his life but was now retired and enjoying his peaceful existence on a property for almost all of his twenty-two years. He now just liked to mooch around the paddock. Then one day out of the blue Riley tried to jump the fence, and in doing so sustained a bad injury to his back. Benjamin, his owner, couldn't understand why he had done this and immediately sought the best treatment for Riley, who recovered quite well—or so Benjamin thought.

A few weeks later, after returning home from work, Benjamin couldn't believe his eyes. Riley was in a traumatised state. He could barely walk and had serious injuries on at least two of his legs and on his chest. Benjamin urgently called the vet but the prognosis wasn't good. In fact the vet couldn't see how, with that level of injury, Riley could possibly recover. To make matters worse, Riley appeared to be in a lot of pain and discomfort. The vet had no alternative but to recommend euthanasia, which Benjamin reluctantly agreed to, but pleaded for a short time alone with Riley first.

He lay down with his big, brave horse and explained why he was saying goodbye. He then solemnly gave the vet permission to do what had to be done, and Riley was suddenly gone. It hit Benjamin very hard as no one knew what had caused the problem.

Benjamin had to deal with the loss of his beloved friend, plus the mystery of his death. He needed to know the truth, so he came to me to get some answers.

When I connected with Riley, I instantly picked up that he was a very strong and proud horse. I felt his inner gentleness and soft heart, and my own heart melted in that moment. I began by asking him what had happened and I was overcome with a deep sadness as he told me his story.

Some years earlier he'd had a female horse companion called Luna. He loved her very much and enjoyed being in her presence. Then one day Riley was moved to another location, and not given time to say goodbye. He missed Luna so much that he tried to immerse himself in training and competitive eventing to help get over his loss. Sadly, but perhaps not surprisingly, during that whole period he never bonded with another horse the way he had with Luna.

When he was retired from eventing his loneliness for companionship became a lot more pressing, although he thought his luck had changed when a new female horse was put into the paddock next to him. Over time he became quite fond of her, but she didn't seem to want a companion in Riley, so Benjamin kept them separate. Riley's longing for a companion overtook him, and hence his impetuous and disastrous jumping of the fence, resulting in his injury.

As Benjamin didn't know the reason for this odd behaviour, he had put Riley back alone in his own paddock after the accident.

When Riley felt he'd recovered quite well and was feeling stronger, he attempted the fence again. Unfortunately his back legs gave way, causing him serious harm. As he went to get up, he found it difficult to stand. In the attempt, he put such a strain on the rest of his body that it resulted in severe damage to his legs and shoulder areas. This was the state that Benjamin found him in.

Riley assured me he'd now found happiness for, as he passed over, Luna was waiting for him. They walked together along the ascending gold path to the other side. He was with her now and forever.

Benjamin was so delighted to have some sort of closure, although he did feel extremely guilty that he'd overlooked Riley's longing for Luna. He knew he was fond of her, but not to that extent. He had had no idea. He exclaimed that had he known, he would have done something about it.

I told Benjamin not to blame himself, as it wasn't possible to be aware of everything that goes on in an animal's life. We have to concentrate on our *own* life also, and none of us is all-knowing.

Benjamin remarked that being able to communicate with animals would certainly create much more clarity and understanding in these relationships—although for him, this information came too late. This is why communication between species is so important. It must be frustrating for the animals to be dealing with a situation and not be able to express it. This is yet another lesson for all of us.

54

Message from beyond the Grave

AS YOU CAN SEE, THE ANIMALS THAT COME INTO OUR LIVES
have much to teach us, and this doesn't stop when they
pass over. Many have shared with me words of wisdom
and encouragement, before and after they have left this
world. Animals work in mysterious ways, as they love us
so unconditionally and come to help and support us on our
life's path. It's nothing short of magic.

Rosemary was heartbroken when her cat, Cherri, passed
away suddenly. She contacted me to get some clarity as to
where she was, and if she was okay. This is what Cherri
had to say:

You have many scars from your past. It is now time to leave
them behind and move forward. I will work with you in the
spirit realms rather than the physical realms, as I have much
work to do here. Don't get in your own way and hold yourself
back from spiritual progress and enlightenment. I am you in

essence, but in cat form, and I know that you recognised this the moment you first saw me. I can only guide you now, as life is a choice, your choice. It is time to follow your dream and be courageous. Trust and believe in yourself. Don't allow excuses to hold you back. Things need to change for new growth to occur. I know you want a sign from me, so watch for the crystal rose quartz. I wish to thank you for the love and glorious moments shared; they will be eternally etched in my soul.

Rosemary said this had given her much peace and closure. Cherri was right about what Rosemary needed to do, as she was living in denial. Just knowing that her beloved Cherri was guiding her through life was the greatest comfort of all.

A few days later Rosemary phoned me. She wanted me to know that one morning she awoke to a noise and looked over to her dresser where there were two rose quartz angels, one on each side of the silver case where she kept Cherri's ashes. Both angels were lying on their sides, as if they'd been knocked over! This was the physical sign she had waited for, as she now knew that Cherri was close by.

If that isn't magic, I don't know what is.

55

Love that Lasts Forever

ANIMALS LOVE TO GIVE US MESSAGES FROM BEYOND THE GRAVE. It's their way of maintaining contact with, and offering guidance to their loved human family. The relationship we have with these much-loved companions is unlike any other we experience. The truth is, this degree of unconditional love and loyalty is a first for many humans, so it is exquisite stuff.

Let me put it this way: our animal friends are silent angels who help us survive the ups and downs of our lives with their constant love, devotion and support. The power of this is unfailing, even in the darkest times. Animals keep us grounded and in touch with a simpler, uncomplicated way of living, and that is both so soothing and reassuring.

When Julie contacted me about Sharna, her Labrador, it had been quite a while since her dog had crossed over. Even though time had passed, she was still finding it difficult to cope without her best friend and companion. Sharna had been such a gentle soul and was never far from Julie's side when on the earth plane. She'd been with Julie for twelve years, sticking by her through the difficulties that come along for each and every one of us.

With Sharna's support, Julie had managed to come through those events resilient, and more at peace than she had ever been. Her devotion to Sharna was so strong she knew there must have been a special reason why they had been together, and why it was so difficult to let her go.

This was Sharna's special message for Julie, conveyed via me:

I was destined to be with you because I am your star sister. We both originated from the same star, and have travelled across time and space together over many lifetimes. We are like two halves that make up the whole. Life here on the earth plane has not been easy for you. I came to lighten your heart, and will continue to do so from these realms. Have faith in who you are and in the decisions you make. We are one heart that beats to the same rhythm. Even though I am no longer on the physical plane, you will still be able to hear and feel me. When you are in a storm of emotion, protect your heart and keep it strong. Grant yourself the time and patience you so willingly give to others. I love you and thank you for all you have given me, and all we have been able to give each other.

Being assigned the privilege to convey that amazing message to Sharna was one of those 'moments' that remind me why I'm on this earth. I dwell so often on the wonder of how, even from the other side, animals can provide us with so much love and support. Their messages are so profound that they can have a life-changing effect on those left behind.

Veronica had such an experience when Rani, her German Shepherd, died. Rani had shared his twelve years of life with Veronica, her husband Richard, and their two sons. Veronica confided to me that she felt Rani had communicated with her a week before he died. He was sitting at her feet looking up at her, and she heard his words in her thoughts. She had never experienced this before.

Rani explained that he had cancer and was very tired. Veronica without hesitation took him to the vet and wanted him examined. After tests were carried out she was astonished when it was confirmed he had cancer. A few days later Rani began bleeding from his mouth and nose and Veronica and Richard were left with no alternative but to assist him by euthanasia. How sad they were, but they did it out of love.

Veronica had never communicated with Rani before and she was bewildered as to why he had chosen that particular time. Why not earlier? Veronica was finding it overwhelmingly difficult to get over the loss of Rani, and she wanted to know if he was all right now, and whether or not she'd done enough with the information he'd given her.

I knew in my heart that Rani had a profound reason for his actions, and when I sat down to connect with him, he was already ready and waiting to speak. He knew exactly why I'd come, and what I was going to ask him. He began by telling me he'd known of his illness for some time, but didn't want Veronica to be shocked at the last minute. But he knew that if he'd told her earlier, there would have been extensive treatments he didn't want. He had to go, and he wanted to thank the family for a wonderful life.

Rani spoke of the two teenage sons, and how different their personalities were. The younger one was quite rebellious and difficult for Veronica and Richard to understand at times. The other was very level-headed, academic and disciplined. Rani wanted to remind them to embrace the differences in people and honour their chosen paths. Ours is not to judge, but to guide. Everyone's adventure is unique unto themselves.

He also asked me to give them the message loud and clear that cancer is really a *human* ailment, which animals contract in order to show that living the human way is flawed. In order to avoid certain cancers, changes must be made.

Rani wanted Veronica to know she has a beautiful soul, which radiated within him; that their strong connection was based on the purity of their love. He put it this way to me: he'd been directing her masculine side, to build strength and vitality. Rani wished to go on supporting Veronica, as he knew she needed strength to move to the next level of her journey. He knew too that she was not at her full potential, always doubting her abilities. Communicating with her about the illness prior to his death, and then having what was said validated by the vet, was the verification she needed to trust in her own instincts now, and in the years ahead.

He also wanted to point out that in the future, her beliefs would be put to the test again and again—and wouldn't always be verified. It would be an exercise in trust.

How wise was Rani! I know in my own life how often I have to take a leap of faith. Yes, it's scary, but whenever I trust my own gut feelings, I usually have a sense of getting closer to the light. Beautiful, clever Rani wanted to convey to Veronica that in order to feel true beauty, you must have a hand in creating it. To become one with the universe is the ultimate goal.

It blew Veronica away when, through me, Rani revealed that her late grandparents had come to greet him as he crossed to the other side. Naturally she was so grateful for this precious message. The communication certainly cleared up many of her questions. It also made her realise that she'd been stifling her spiritual journey with family commitments—now it was time to fly, to move forward on her own individual path. In return for these gifts from Rani, she promised him she'd use his strength and support to fulfill her destiny.

Connecting with animals in spirit has always been a profound experience for me. As an intuitive, I have the rare privilege of not only hearing these animal spirits when they speak of their philosophies, but also of experiencing the visions and the energy they communicate. I have been enriched, over and over again, and I honour and bless the animals for granting me these luminous insights.

Epilogue

It's All about Loving Us

FROM THE INSTANT I WAS BORN UNTIL NOW, MY LOVE FOR animals has run very deep, as this book has shown you. There have been so many moments in my life where just to look at animals has brought tears to my eyes. These have mostly been tears of pure joy, but some have been caused by sadness when I've heard about cruelty to these amazing animal beings. I see beauty in animals that can be difficult to describe. I am in awe of the unconditional sense of love they offer, along with the way they help us become remarkable people.

Lives are changed by animals. They literally help us to open our hearts without fear—not only to ourselves, but to others. They have touched me in a way that has transformed my thinking about who I want to be. There have been dozens and dozens of special animals for me, with dearest Beau being the standout. I've been blessed in that regard. Animals have taught me so many precious truths.

While working with another professional communicator in the United States, I learnt an unusual lesson in trust. This memorable experience happened with Solstice, an exceptionally large, grey Warmblood Thoroughbred cross. I went up to the stables where he and two other horses were agisted. As I walked up to the paddock and approached the horses, there was already a stillness from the slow, deliberate movement of the horses' grazing. Finding a restful spot out of the way of the horses seemed ideal, and so I flopped down on the soft, moist grass, partially shaded by large oak trees. I didn't want to observe, but to become part of this peaceful scene. As far as I could tell, the horses were oblivious to my presence, or so I thought.

Solstice was a likely choice for my telepathic conversation as he was strong and handsome, and he greatly appealed to me. I have to admit there was already a connection between us from the moment our eyes met. He appeared to be the leader of the others. Sitting cross-legged on the ground quite some distance from Solstice and with my eyes closed, I was ready to communicate with him.

A couple of minutes passed and I heard a munching of grass and the thud of a hoof. It sounded very close and made me feel somewhat nervous to sense that such a big animal was so near. I had to open my eyes to reassure myself he was still at a safe distance from me. Yes, he was a few metres away, so I tried to tell myself everything was fine—even though I could feel the rapid beating of my heart.

I closed my eyes rather nervously and attempted to resume my telepathic communication when I received the words, *I won't hurt you, don't be afraid.* What was going on! With my eyes firmly shut, I still believed that Solstice hadn't managed to silently creep up beside me, given his size, and I told him that. But those munching and thud sounds were so close that I finally opened my eyes again, only to find him walking and eating the grass only centimetres from me. He was literally towering over me. This was too much for me to handle. I had to get up and go and sit on an old plastic chair nearby, where it felt safer. I resumed my communication from there, and he kept his distance after that.

A year later, I returned to do some more work with the horses for my telepathic development. I walked straight up to the top paddock to see Solstice, greeting him warmly. He replied, *You've come back.* I felt I'd got to know him quite well, so I was far more relaxed around him this time.

Solstice had the type of personality that made him want to be noticed for his strong persona and intelligence as an individual, rather than just for his species type. Even though not outwardly affectionate with most people, I knew he had a deeply loving heart. I also knew he felt this closeness could detract from his purpose of strength in the horse hierarchy. Solstice needed to feel he had freedom over his life: he wanted to make his own decisions.

I told him he mustn't play that creeping-up trick on me again and just to make sure that he couldn't, I sat on an incline under a very low-branched tree, where he could hardly see me. As I closed my eyes ready to communicate, I heard him approach, so I opened my eyes with confidence, knowing the branches prevented him from getting too close. To my utter amazement, he was crouching down on his hocks, practically crawling to get under the tree. He kept communicating to me, conveying that he wouldn't harm me. After he made several attempts to reach me, I thought if he was that desperate to get close, then maybe I should let him. So I moved out into the open paddock, sat cross-legged and told him to go ahead and do what it was he wanted to do for me.

Solstice, with his powerful stature, walked right behind me very slowly, just contacting his hoofs very lightly on my body as he went past. I heaved a big sigh of relief: he hadn't hurt me; quite the opposite, Solstice had been so gentle. As he continued to walk away, I looked around at him and he looked around at me and he told me he'd never hurt me, because he was my Pegasus!

Feeling such love for him, I got straight up, ran over and hugged him. What he'd just said had brought tears to my eyes because, as a child, I'd always dreamt of a white horse with wings. This magnificent white horse would fly down to collect me on his back and take me off to a magical land. Solstice had done just that; he'd taken me to that magical place of animals.

Telepathic communication really does change relationships and understanding. With the guidance of animals, we can learn the truth of who we are, and why we're here. I have no doubt they come into our lives to support us and to spur us on to grow, personally and spiritually.

Acknowledgements

THIS BOOK HAS BEEN INSPIRED BY MY EXPERIENCE OF DISCOVERING the wonders of communicating with animals in their silent language and observing the many people who have come to me for help now having a greater understanding of their animals.

The mere translation of the words of their animals has brought incalculable joy to hundreds of humans, while for me, it has been a great privilege getting to know and understand all of their amazing animals.

Although it has been a continuing adventure, I must say that I have treasured everything so far, and will always be so incredibly grateful for the experiences. Thank you! Thank you to all the animals who have touched my life in some way and shared their wisdom.

Writing this book was such a journey of personal and spiritual discovery—discovering the depth of my own thoughts and having true belief in what I was writing and sharing with the rest of the world. The journey began with a cat named Beau, who showed me that if you are not doing what makes your heart sing then you are on the wrong path. Without you Beau and the extreme love between us I would never have set off to be a Voice of the Animals. The inspiration of this book and its inception I believe began the day you came into my life.

Mattie and Shea, I can't thank you enough for your continued support, unconditional love and belief in me through this whole process. Mattie you just knew how to sit on the keyboard of my computer when I needed a break. Shea you always made it very clear when it was time to go to bed with your very special vocal reminder.

Savannah, you relentlessly sat beside my computer on the desk through the many hours of creation, so I would not do this alone. Akeira, you were forever in my face reminding me that taking a walk right now would clear my mind and allow for greater clarity for my words.

Slasher, my beloved childhood dog, you shaped my loving memories of animals as a child. Cimmeron, my first cat, you were so unusual in your antics I thought all cats could catch objects in their paws. Winston, my wonderful companion, you were always at my side in some of the hardest moments of my life. The beautiful Chinchilla Misty, you became such a close friend when I embarked out on my own in life. You have all been such an integral part in the roots of my relationships and understanding of the beauty of animals sharing people's lives.

My support and encouragement has also come from the human species. I wish to thank my husband Peter for his amazing understanding as I embarked on this new world of animal communication. Without your support it would have been extremely difficult for me to have continued with such ease and persistence. Indeed you are a man of great insight.

I wish to thank my mum Evelyn, and sisters Vicki and Rebecca, as none of you ever stopped believing I could do anything I set out to do. Some of this book was written in our family home and you gave me the space and support I so needed.

My wonderful friend Max, you are such a unique individual and an integral part of my work. An inspiration and mentor you have always been at my side through the process of this book and my life as an animal communicator. Thanks for being my best friend when I needed it most.

Karen, my friend and colleague in much of my spiritual work, you always encouraged me to speak my truth; to follow my beliefs and insights and take them to new levels. I feel I have done so in this book.

Charlene, you and I share a great love of animals and ours is a friendship that has grown so beautifully over time. You have always supported me in this work but most of all as a person. Your belief and trust in me is unsurpassed.

A big thank you to Maggie, my publisher, you are amazing. You have a way of making writing a book so simple, even when you think it is at its most difficult stage. You pulled me through all the way to make sure the world knows how wonderful animals really are.

Thank you also to all my clients and their animals who provided me with the most amazing stories to tell. Without them there is no book or enlightening tales of the deep love and heartwarming relationships between people and animals.

Of course, last but not least, to all the animals who are or ever have been on this planet sharing their lives with us, a big thank you for being our teachers. Sharing your joy and love and making the world a better place; making us better people. Thank you for making so many dreams come true!